ATS-32 ADMISSION TEST SERIES

This is your
PASSBOOK for...

Dental Hygiene Aptitude Test (DHAT)

Test Preparation Study Guide
Questions & Answers

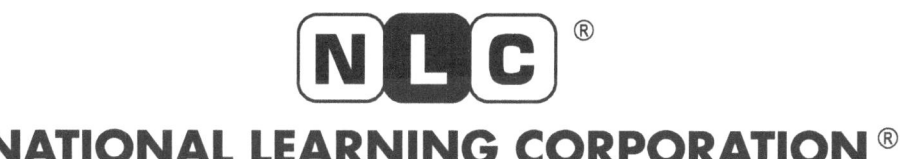

NATIONAL LEARNING CORPORATION®

COPYRIGHT NOTICE

This book is SOLELY intended for, is sold ONLY to, and its use is RESTRICTED to individual, bona fide applicants or candidates who qualify by virtue of having seriously filed applications for appropriate license, certificate, professional and/or promotional advancement, higher school matriculation, scholarship, or other legitimate requirements of education and/or governmental authorities.

This book is NOT intended for use, class instruction, tutoring, training, duplication, copying, reprinting, excerption, or adaptation, etc., by:

1) Other publishers
2) Proprietors and/or Instructors of "Coaching" and/or Preparatory Courses
3) Personnel and/or Training Divisions of commercial, industrial, and governmental organizations
4) Schools, colleges, or universities and/or their departments and staffs, including teachers and other personnel
5) Testing Agencies or Bureaus
6) Study groups which seek by the purchase of a single volume to copy and/or duplicate and/or adapt this material for use by the group as a whole without having purchased individual volumes for each of the members of the group
7) Et al.

Such persons would be in violation of appropriate Federal and State statutes.

PROVISION OF LICENSING AGREEMENTS – Recognized educational, commercial, industrial, and governmental institutions and organizations, and others legitimately engaged in educational pursuits, including training, testing, and measurement activities, may address request for a licensing agreement to the copyright owners, who will determine whether, and under what conditions, including fees and charges, the materials in this book may be used them. In other words, a licensing facility exists for the legitimate use of the material in this book on other than an individual basis. However, it is asseverated and affirmed here that the material in this book CANNOT be used without the receipt of the express permission of such a licensing agreement from the Publishers. Inquiries re licensing should be addressed to the company, attention rights and permissions department.

All rights reserved, including the right of reproduction in whole or in part, in any form or by any means, electronic or mechanical, including photocopying, recording, or by any information storage and retrieval system, without permission in writing from the Publisher.

Copyright © 2024 by
National Learning Corporation

212 Michael Drive, Syosset, NY 11791
(516) 921-8888 • www.passbooks.com
E-mail: info@passbooks.com

PUBLISHED IN THE UNITED STATES OF AMERICA

PASSBOOK® SERIES

THE *PASSBOOK® SERIES* has been created to prepare applicants and candidates for the ultimate academic battlefield – the examination room.

At some time in our lives, each and every one of us may be required to take an examination – for validation, matriculation, admission, qualification, registration, certification, or licensure.

Based on the assumption that every applicant or candidate has met the basic formal educational standards, has taken the required number of courses, and read the necessary texts, the *PASSBOOK® SERIES* furnishes the one special preparation which may assure passing with confidence, instead of failing with insecurity. Examination questions – together with answers – are furnished as the basic vehicle for study so that the mysteries of the examination and its compounding difficulties may be eliminated or diminished by a sure method.

This book is meant to help you pass your examination provided that you qualify and are serious in your objective.

The entire field is reviewed through the huge store of content information which is succinctly presented through a provocative and challenging approach – the question-and-answer method.

A climate of success is established by furnishing the correct answers at the end of each test.

You soon learn to recognize types of questions, forms of questions, and patterns of questioning. You may even begin to anticipate expected outcomes.

You perceive that many questions are repeated or adapted so that you can gain acute insights, which may enable you to score many sure points.

You learn how to confront new questions, or types of questions, and to attack them confidently and work out the correct answers.

You note objectives and emphases, and recognize pitfalls and dangers, so that you may make positive educational adjustments.

Moreover, you are kept fully informed in relation to new concepts, methods, practices, and directions in the field.

You discover that you are actually taking the examination all the time: you are preparing for the examination by "taking" an examination, not by reading extraneous and/or supererogatory textbooks.

In short, this PASSBOOK®, used directedly, should be an important factor in helping you to pass your test.

DENTAL HYGIENE APTITUDE TEST (DHAT)

GENERAL

Graduation from a college preparatory curriculum of an accredited secondary school is the minimum educational requirement for admission to a dental hygiene program. Some dental hygiene programs require one or two years of college education, with specified courses for admission. Applicants are expected to have above-average grades, and interest in, and aptitude for, the study and practice of dental hygiene. Some schools have additional admission requirements.

A candidate seeking admission to a dental hygiene school should secure information on specific admission requirements directly from the school. It is important to determine whether the Dental Hygiene Aptitude Test or other tests are required and to arrange for examination well in advance of the deadline for submitting admission application and test scores. The number of students admitted to a dental hygiene program is limited; therefore, it is important to observe dates for filing application.

DENTAL HYGIENE CURRICULUM

Accredited dental hygiene programs include a minimum of two years of college education leading to a certificate, diploma, or associate degree. Four-year baccalaureate degree programs admit students in the first, second or third year of college, depending upon the curriculum of the particular school.

Courses in basic sciences, dental sciences, dental hygiene and liberal arts are included in the curriculum. The dental hygiene student has learning experiences in the classroom, laboratory and clinic.

ABOUT THE EXAMINATION

The tests in the Dental Hygiene Aptitude Testing Program measure abilities in the following areas:

1. *Numerical Ability* – Ability to reason with numbers, and to deal intelligently with quantitative materials; skill in fundamental arithmetic processes including basic knowledge of decimals, fractions, and percentages

2. *Science* – General background knowledge of biology, chemistry, and physics

3. *Verbal* – General knowledge of English, particularly widely used vocabulary

4. *Study-Reading* – Ability to read, organize, analyze, and remember new information; ability to comprehend thoroughly when reading scientific information

HOW TO TAKE A TEST

You have studied long, hard and conscientiously.

With your official admission card in hand, and your heart pounding, you have been admitted to the examination room.

You note that there are several hundred other applicants in the examination room waiting to take the same test.

They all appear to be equally well prepared.

You know that nothing but your best effort will suffice. The "moment of truth" is at hand: you now have to demonstrate objectively, in writing, your knowledge of content and your understanding of subject matter.

You are fighting the most important battle of your life—to pass and/or score high on an examination which will determine your career and provide the economic basis for your livelihood.

What extra, special things should you know and should you do in taking the examination?

I. YOU MUST PASS AN EXAMINATION

A. WHAT EVERY CANDIDATE SHOULD KNOW
Examination applicants often ask us for help in preparing for the written test. What can I study in advance? What kinds of questions will be asked? How will the test be given? How will the papers be graded?

B. HOW ARE EXAMS DEVELOPED?
Examinations are carefully written by trained technicians who are specialists in the field known as "psychological measurement," in consultation with recognized authorities in the field of work that the test will cover. These experts recommend the subject matter areas or skills to be tested; only those knowledges or skills important to your success on the job are included. The most reliable books and source materials available are used as references. Together, the experts and technicians judge the difficulty level of the questions.
Test technicians know how to phrase questions so that the problem is clearly stated. Their ethics do not permit "trick" or "catch" questions. Questions may have been tried out on sample groups, or subjected to statistical analysis, to determine their usefulness.
Written tests are often used in combination with performance tests, ratings of training and experience, and oral interviews. All of these measures combine to form the best-known means of finding the right person for the right job.

II. HOW TO PASS THE WRITTEN TEST

A. BASIC STEPS

1) Study the announcement

How, then, can you know what subjects to study? Our best answer is: "Learn as much as possible about the class of positions for which you've applied." The exam will test the knowledge, skills and abilities needed to do the work.

Your most valuable source of information about the position you want is the official exam announcement. This announcement lists the training and experience qualifications. Check these standards and apply only if you come reasonably close to meeting them. Many jurisdictions preview the written test in the exam announcement by including a section called "Knowledge and Abilities Required," "Scope of the Examination," or some similar heading. Here you will find out specifically what fields will be tested.

2) Choose appropriate study materials

If the position for which you are applying is technical or advanced, you will read more advanced, specialized material. If you are already familiar with the basic principles of your field, elementary textbooks would waste your time. Concentrate on advanced textbooks and technical periodicals. Think through the concepts and review difficult problems in your field.

These are all general sources. You can get more ideas on your own initiative, following these leads. For example, training manuals and publications of the government agency which employs workers in your field can be useful, particularly for technical and professional positions. A letter or visit to the government department involved may result in more specific study suggestions, and certainly will provide you with a more definite idea of the exact nature of the position you are seeking.

3) Study this book!

III. KINDS OF TESTS

Tests are used for purposes other than measuring knowledge and ability to perform specified duties. For some positions, it is equally important to test ability to make adjustments to new situations or to profit from training. In others, basic mental abilities not dependent on information are essential. Questions which test these things may not appear as pertinent to the duties of the position as those which test for knowledge and information. Yet they are often highly important parts of a fair examination. For very general questions, it is almost impossible to help you direct your study efforts. What we can do is to point out some of the more common of these general abilities needed in public service positions and describe some typical questions.

1) General information

Broad, general information has been found useful for predicting job success in some kinds of work. This is tested in a variety of ways, from vocabulary lists to questions about current events. Basic background in some field of work, such as sociology or economics, may be sampled in a group of questions. Often these are principles which have become familiar to most persons through exposure rather than through formal training. It is difficult to advise you how to study for these questions; being alert to the world around you is our best suggestion.

2) Verbal ability

An example of an ability needed in many positions is verbal or language ability. Verbal ability is, in brief, the ability to use and understand words. Vocabulary and grammar tests are typical measures of this ability. Reading comprehension or paragraph interpretation questions are common in many kinds of civil service tests. You are given a paragraph of written material and asked to find its central meaning.

IV. KINDS OF QUESTIONS

1. Multiple-choice Questions

Most popular of the short-answer questions is the "multiple choice" or "best answer" question. It can be used, for example, to test for factual knowledge, ability to solve problems or judgment in meeting situations found at work.

A multiple-choice question is normally one of three types:
- It can begin with an incomplete statement followed by several possible endings. You are to find the one ending which best completes the statement, although some of the others may not be entirely wrong.
- It can also be a complete statement in the form of a question which is answered by choosing one of the statements listed.
- It can be in the form of a problem – again you select the best answer.

Here is an example of a multiple-choice question with a discussion which should give you some clues as to the method for choosing the right answer:

When an employee has a complaint about his assignment, the action which will best help him overcome his difficulty is to
- A. discuss his difficulty with his coworkers
- B. take the problem to the head of the organization
- C. take the problem to the person who gave him the assignment
- D. say nothing to anyone about his complaint

In answering this question, you should study each of the choices to find which is best. Consider choice "A" – Certainly an employee may discuss his complaint with fellow employees, but no change or improvement can result, and the complaint remains unresolved. Choice "B" is a poor choice since the head of the organization probably does not know what assignment you have been given, and taking your problem to him is known as "going over the head" of the supervisor. The supervisor, or person who made the assignment, is the person who can clarify it or correct any injustice. Choice "C" is, therefore, correct. To say nothing, as in choice "D," is unwise. Supervisors have and interest in knowing the problems employees are facing, and the employee is seeking a solution to his problem.

2. True/False

3. Matching Questions

Matching an answer from a column of choices within another column.

V. RECORDING YOUR ANSWERS

Computer terminals are used more and more today for many different kinds of exams.

For an examination with very few applicants, you may be told to record your answers in the test booklet itself. Separate answer sheets are much more common. If this separate answer sheet is to be scored by machine – and this is often the case – it is highly important that you mark your answers correctly in order to get credit.

VI. BEFORE THE TEST

YOUR PHYSICAL CONDITION IS IMPORTANT

If you are not well, you can't do your best work on tests. If you are half asleep, you can't do your best either. Here are some tips:

1) Get about the same amount of sleep you usually get. Don't stay up all night before the test, either partying or worrying—DON'T DO IT!
2) If you wear glasses, be sure to wear them when you go to take the test. This goes for hearing aids, too.
3) If you have any physical problems that may keep you from doing your best, be sure to tell the person giving the test. If you are sick or in poor health, you relay cannot do your best on any test. You can always come back and take the test some other time.

Common sense will help you find procedures to follow to get ready for an examination. Too many of us, however, overlook these sensible measures. Indeed, nervousness and fatigue have been found to be the most serious reasons why applicants fail to do their best on civil service tests. Here is a list of reminders:

- Begin your preparation early – Don't wait until the last minute to go scurrying around for books and materials or to find out what the position is all about.
- Prepare continuously – An hour a night for a week is better than an all-night cram session. This has been definitely established. What is more, a night a week for a month will return better dividends than crowding your study into a shorter period of time.
- Locate the place of the exam – You have been sent a notice telling you when and where to report for the examination. If the location is in a different town or otherwise unfamiliar to you, it would be well to inquire the best route and learn something about the building.
- Relax the night before the test – Allow your mind to rest. Do not study at all that night. Plan some mild recreation or diversion; then go to bed early and get a good night's sleep.
- Get up early enough to make a leisurely trip to the place for the test – This way unforeseen events, traffic snarls, unfamiliar buildings, etc. will not upset you.
- Dress comfortably – A written test is not a fashion show. You will be known by number and not by name, so wear something comfortable.
- Leave excess paraphernalia at home – Shopping bags and odd bundles will get in your way. You need bring only the items mentioned in the official notice you received; usually everything you need is provided. Do not bring reference books to the exam. They will only confuse those last minutes and be taken away from you when in the test room.

- Arrive somewhat ahead of time – If because of transportation schedules you must get there very early, bring a newspaper or magazine to take your mind off yourself while waiting.
- Locate the examination room – When you have found the proper room, you will be directed to the seat or part of the room where you will sit. Sometimes you are given a sheet of instructions to read while you are waiting. Do not fill out any forms until you are told to do so; just read them and be prepared.
- Relax and prepare to listen to the instructions
- If you have any physical problem that may keep you from doing your best, be sure to tell the test administrator. If you are sick or in poor health, you really cannot do your best on the exam. You can come back and take the test some other time.

VII. AT THE TEST

The day of the test is here and you have the test booklet in your hand. The temptation to get going is very strong. Caution! There is more to success than knowing the right answers. You must know how to identify your papers and understand variations in the type of short-answer question used in this particular examination. Follow these suggestions for maximum results from your efforts:

1) Cooperate with the monitor

The test administrator has a duty to create a situation in which you can be as much at ease as possible. He will give instructions, tell you when to begin, check to see that you are marking your answer sheet correctly, and so on. He is not there to guard you, although he will see that your competitors do not take unfair advantage. He wants to help you do your best.

2) Listen to all instructions

Don't jump the gun! Wait until you understand all directions. In most civil service tests you get more time than you need to answer the questions. So don't be in a hurry. Read each word of instructions until you clearly understand the meaning. Study the examples, listen to all announcements and follow directions. Ask questions if you do not understand what to do.

3) Identify your papers

Civil service exams are usually identified by number only. You will be assigned a number; you must not put your name on your test papers. Be sure to copy your number correctly. Since more than one exam may be given, copy your exact examination title.

4) Plan your time

Unless you are told that a test is a "speed" or "rate of work" test, speed itself is usually not important. Time enough to answer all the questions will be provided, but this does not mean that you have all day. An overall time limit has been set. Divide the total time (in minutes) by the number of questions to determine the approximate time you have for each question.

5) Do not linger over difficult questions

If you come across a difficult question, mark it with a paper clip (useful to have along) and come back to it when you have been through the booklet. One caution if you do this – be sure to skip a number on your answer sheet as well. Check often to be sure that you have not lost your place and that you are marking in the row numbered the same as the question you are answering.

6) Read the questions

Be sure you know what the question asks! Many capable people are unsuccessful because they failed to read the questions correctly.

7) Answer all questions

Unless you have been instructed that a penalty will be deducted for incorrect answers, it is better to guess than to omit a question.

8) Speed tests

It is often better NOT to guess on speed tests. It has been found that on timed tests people are tempted to spend the last few seconds before time is called in marking answers at random – without even reading them – in the hope of picking up a few extra points. To discourage this practice, the instructions may warn you that your score will be "corrected" for guessing. That is, a penalty will be applied. The incorrect answers will be deducted from the correct ones, or some other penalty formula will be used.

9) Review your answers

If you finish before time is called, go back to the questions you guessed or omitted to give them further thought. Review other answers if you have time.

10) Return your test materials

If you are ready to leave before others have finished or time is called, take ALL your materials to the monitor and leave quietly. Never take any test material with you. The monitor can discover whose papers are not complete, and taking a test booklet may be grounds for disqualification.

VIII. EXAMINATION TECHNIQUES

1) Read the general instructions carefully. These are usually printed on the first page of the exam booklet. As a rule, these instructions refer to the timing of the examination; the fact that you should not start work until the signal and must stop work at a signal, etc. If there are any special instructions, such as a choice of questions to be answered, make sure that you note this instruction carefully.

2) When you are ready to start work on the examination, that is as soon as the signal has been given, read the instructions to each question booklet, underline any key words or phrases, such as least, best, outline, describe and the like. In this way you will tend to answer as requested rather than discover on reviewing your paper that you listed without describing, that you selected the worst choice rather than the best choice, etc.

3) If the examination is of the objective or multiple-choice type – that is, each question will also give a series of possible answers: A, B, C or D, and you are called upon to select the best answer and write the letter next to that answer on your answer paper – it is advisable to start answering each question in turn. There may be anywhere from 50 to 100 such questions in the three or four hours allotted and you can see how much time would be taken if you read through all the questions before beginning to answer any. Furthermore, if you

come across a question or group of questions which you know would be difficult to answer, it would undoubtedly affect your handling of all the other questions.

4) If the examination is of the essay type and contains but a few questions, it is a moot point as to whether you should read all the questions before starting to answer any one. Of course, if you are given a choice – say five out of seven and the like – then it is essential to read all the questions so you can eliminate the two that are most difficult. If, however, you are asked to answer all the questions, there may be danger in trying to answer the easiest one first because you may find that you will spend too much time on it. The best technique is to answer the first question, then proceed to the second, etc.

5) Time your answers. Before the exam begins, write down the time it started, then add the time allowed for the examination and write down the time it must be completed, then divide the time available somewhat as follows:
    - If 3-1/2 hours are allowed, that would be 210 minutes. If you have 80 objective-type questions, that would be an average of 2-1/2 minutes per question. Allow yourself no more than 2 minutes per question, or a total of 160 minutes, which will permit about 50 minutes to review.
    - If for the time allotment of 210 minutes there are 7 essay questions to answer, that would average about 30 minutes a question. Give yourself only 25 minutes per question so that you have about 35 minutes to review.

6) The most important instruction is to read each question and make sure you know what is wanted. The second most important instruction is to time yourself properly so that you answer every question. The third most important instruction is to answer every question. Guess if you have to but include something for each question. Remember that you will receive no credit for a blank and will probably receive some credit if you write something in answer to an essay question. If you guess a letter – say "B" for a multiple-choice question – you may have guessed right. If you leave a blank as an answer to a multiple-choice question, the examiners may respect your feelings but it will not add a point to your score. Some exams may penalize you for wrong answers, so in such cases only, you may not want to guess unless you have some basis for your answer.

7) Suggestions
    a. Objective-type questions
        1. Examine the question booklet for proper sequence of pages and questions
        2. Read all instructions carefully
        3. Skip any question which seems too difficult; return to it after all other questions have been answered
        4. Apportion your time properly; do not spend too much time on any single question or group of questions
        5. Note and underline key words – all, most, fewest, least, best, worst, same, opposite, etc.
        6. Pay particular attention to negatives
        7. Note unusual option, e.g., unduly long, short, complex, different or similar in content to the body of the question
        8. Observe the use of "hedging" words – probably, may, most likely, etc.

9. Make sure that your answer is put next to the same number as the question
10. Do not second-guess unless you have good reason to believe the second answer is definitely more correct
11. Cross out original answer if you decide another answer is more accurate; do not erase until you are ready to hand your paper in
12. Answer all questions; guess unless instructed otherwise
13. Leave time for review

b. Essay questions
1. Read each question carefully
2. Determine exactly what is wanted. Underline key words or phrases.
3. Decide on outline or paragraph answer
4. Include many different points and elements unless asked to develop any one or two points or elements
5. Show impartiality by giving pros and cons unless directed to select one side only
6. Make and write down any assumptions you find necessary to answer the questions
7. Watch your English, grammar, punctuation and choice of words
8. Time your answers; don't crowd material

8) Answering the essay question

Most essay questions can be answered by framing the specific response around several key words or ideas. Here are a few such key words or ideas:

M's: manpower, materials, methods, money, management
P's: purpose, program, policy, plan, procedure, practice, problems, pitfalls, personnel, public relations

a. Six basic steps in handling problems:
1. Preliminary plan and background development
2. Collect information, data and facts
3. Analyze and interpret information, data and facts
4. Analyze and develop solutions as well as make recommendations
5. Prepare report and sell recommendations
6. Install recommendations and follow up effectiveness

b. Pitfalls to avoid
1. Taking things for granted – A statement of the situation does not necessarily imply that each of the elements is necessarily true; for example, a complaint may be invalid and biased so that all that can be taken for granted is that a complaint has been registered
2. Considering only one side of a situation – Wherever possible, indicate several alternatives and then point out the reasons you selected the best one
3. Failing to indicate follow up – Whenever your answer indicates action on your part, make certain that you will take proper follow-up action to see how successful your recommendations, procedures or actions turn out to be
4. Taking too long in answering any single question – Remember to time your answers properly

EXAMINATION SECTION

EXAMINATION SECTION
TEST 1

DIRECTIONS: Each question or incomplete statement is followed by several suggested answers or completions. Select the one that BEST answers the question or completes the statement. *PRINT THE LETTER OF THE CORRECT ANSWER IN THE SPACE AT THE RIGHT.*

1. An experiment was conducted in which juice was extracted from an infected tobacco plant and passes through a porcelain filter.
   When this juice was brought into contact with a healthy tobacco plant and caused the same disease, the experiment led to the discovery of

   A. bacteria
   B. protozoa
   C. viruses
   D. cancer cells

2. A genetic variation in which a new gene takes over the locus of the old is referred to as a(n)

   A. aberration
   B. mutation
   C. translocation
   D. deficiency

3. When black, rough-coated guinea pigs, hybrid for both color and texture of coat, are crossed, some of their offspring are white, smooth-coated guinea pigs.
   This is a classic illustration of the law of

   A. independent assortment
   B. dominance
   C. linkage
   D. segregation

4. Which one of the following receptors is INCORRECTLY paired with the structure in which it is found?

   A. Taste bud - Tongue
   B. Rod - Retina
   C. Cone - Retina
   D. Proprioceptor - Nasal epithelium

5. A gland which acts both as a duct gland as well as a ductless gland is the

   A. thyroid
   B. adrenal
   C. parathyroid
   D. pancreas

6. A vitamin formerly thought to be a simple compound but now known to be a complex of at least ten separate vitamins is vitamin

   A. A
   B. B
   C. C
   D. D

7. Of the following nutrients, the one which is absorbed by the lymph, rather than by the blood in the capillaries, is

   A. amino acids
   B. fatty acids
   C. glucose
   D. water

8. A person of type AB blood should be given a transfusion

   A. only from O and AB
   B. only from AB and A
   C. only from AB and B
   D. from either O, A, B, or AB

9. A classic study on human gastric digestion was performed by

   A. Beaumont   B. Schleiden   C. Pavlov   D. Banting

10. The nervous system is derived from

    A. ectoderm
    B. mesoderm
    C. endoderm
    D. a combination of endoderm and ectoderm

11. Which one of the following series is in the CORRECT sequence?

    A. Fertilized egg, cleavage, blastula, gastrula
    B. Blastula, fertilized egg, gastrula, cleavage
    C. Blastula, cleavage, gastrula, fertilized egg
    D. Fertilized egg, blastula, cleavage, gastrula

12. Which one of the following statements regarding plant hormones is NOT true?

    A. Despite much research, auxins have thus far not been synthesized.
    B. The auxins from an oat coleoptile can be absorbed on a block of agar and used for further experimentation.
    C. Auxins accelerate lengthwise growth in the stem.
    D. Auxins retard lengthwise growth in the root.

13. In a woody stem, all growth results from the activity of the

    A. cambium   B. phloem   C. pith   D. xylem

14. Which one of the following pairs is INCORRECTLY matched?

    A. Strawberry - eyes   B. Raspberry - layers
    C. Onion - bulbs   D. Potato - tubers

15. It was a relatively simple task for Mendel to secure pure lines in the garden pea since in nature it is _____ pollinated.

    A. wind   B. insect   C. water   D. self

16. Respiration in plants is

    A. similar to respiration in animals and takes place at all times
    B. similar to respiration in animals and takes place only when the plant is not carrying on photosynthesis
    C. different from respiration in animals and takes place at all times
    D. different from respiration in animals and takes place only when the plant is not carrying on photo-synthesis

17. Modern research indicates that photosynthesis consists

    A. only of rapid light reactions
    B. only of slow light reactions
    C. only of a dark reaction
    D. of a light reaction followed by a dark reaction

18. Cells obtain energy quickly through 18.____

    A. photosynthesis
    B. oxidation of glucose
    C. hydrolysis of ATP
    D. osmosis

19. Which one of the following statements with regard to enzymes is NOT true? 19.____

    A. Enzymes are organic catalysts produced by living cells
    B. Enzymes are specific, frequently acting only upon a single substrate.
    C. An enzyme can accelerate a specific reaction in only one direction.
    D. Enzymes have a protein component.

20. A reduction division takes place 20.____

    A. only in animal cells during mitosis
    B. only in plant cells during mitosis
    C. in both plant and animal cells during mitosis
    D. in both plant and animal cells during meiosis

21. The essential determiner of heredity in every living cell is a substance known as 21.____

    A. DNA   B. ACTH   C. 2-4D   D. ATP

22. If the number of protons in the nucleus of each atom is the same as the number in every other atom, the substance is 22.____

    A. inert
    B. an active non-metal
    C. amphoteric
    D. an element

23. Of the following atomic particles, the LIGHTEST in weight is the 23.____

    A. proton
    B. electron
    C. alpha particle
    D. neutron

24. The PRINCIPAL difference between a mixture and a chemical compound is that a 24.____

    A. mixture is always heterogeneous in composition
    B. mixture does not contain chemical substances
    C. compound is always of definite composition
    D. compound is more easily separated into its constituent parts

25. Boiling is an effective method of purifying water that contains 25.____

    A. soluble organic impurities
    B. bacteria and dissolved gases
    C. insoluble inorganic impurities
    D. soluble organic impurities and bacteria

KEY (CORRECT ANSWERS)

1.	C	11.	A
2.	B	12.	A
3.	A	13.	A
4.	D	14.	A
5.	D	15.	D
6.	B	16.	A
7.	B	17.	D
8.	D	18.	C
9.	A	19.	C
10.	A	20.	D

21. A
22. D
23. B
24. C
25. B

TEST 2

DIRECTIONS: Each question or incomplete statement is followed by several suggested answers or completions. Select the one that BEST answers the question or completes the statement. *PRINT THE LETTER OF THE CORRECT ANSWER IN THE SPACE AT THE RIGHT.*

1. An inexpensive, readily available raw material for the chemical manufacture of washing soda, hydrochloric acid and chlorine, is

    A. NaCl
    B. Na_2CO_3
    C. HCl
    D. $Na_2CO_3 \cdot 10H_2O$

    1.____

2. About 75% of the air by weight is

    A. carbon dioxide
    B. argon
    C. oxygen
    D. nitrogen

    2.____

3. Argon gas is used to fill tungsten filament electric light bulbs because it

    A. supports the combustion of the filament
    B. offers less resistance to the flow of current than nitrogen
    C. is inert and slows the evaporation of the filament
    D. is less expensive than pure oxygen

    3.____

4. The number of sub atomic particles that have been identi-fied are

    A. ten
    B. twenty-five
    C. fifty
    D. one hundred

    4.____

5. In ordinary chemical reactions, atoms combine with each other when

    A. electrons are transferred from one atom to another
    B. nuclear particles are shared
    C. one atom loses protons gained by the other
    D. the transfer of particles produces ions with no electrical charge

    5.____

6. Adenine, thymine, cytosine, and guanine are ALL

    A. chemical names for common vitamins
    B. units that constitute the genetic code of DNA
    C. important hormones
    D. enzymes active in digestion

    6.____

7. A gas distributed commercially in solid form for use as a refrigerant is

    A. chlorine
    B. carbon dioxide
    C. argon
    D. nitrogen

    7.____

8. Paraffin wax used to make candles is obtained commercially by

    A. the cracking of kerosene
    B. the hydrogenation of fuel oil
    C. the fractional distillation of crude oil
    D. polymerization of pure hydrocarbons

    8.____

9. The E.M.F. that pushes electrons through an electrical circuit is measured in

    A. ohms   B. volts   C. coulombs   D. amperes

10. The north pole of a compass needle will often point slightly away from true north because the

    A. compass needle does not line up with the magnetic lines of force of the earth
    B. North Star is not an accurate reference point for determining true north
    C. magnetic pole and the geographic pole of the earth do not coincide
    D. position of the geographic North Pole is not definite

11. If 1 quart of water at 100° C is added to 1 gallon of water at 0° C, the number of calories gained by the colder water as compared with the number of calories lost by the warmer water is as

    A. 1:1   B. 1:4   C. 4:1   D. 0.25:1

12. A bobsled track is banked at the turns in order to over-come

    A. drag
    B. centrifugal force
    C. friction
    D. gravity

13. In Einstein's formula $E = MC^2$, the factor E = energy, M = mass, and C represents

    A. the speed of light
    B. Hooke's constant
    C. the Lorentz transformation factor
    D. Planck's constant

14. A solid cube will float in water if the

    A. weight of the water it displaces is less than the weight of the cube
    B. water density is greater than the density of the cube
    C. water has expanded due to heating
    D. difference in weight between the cube and an equal volume of water is less than 1 gm.

15. A block will slide with uniform velocity down an inclined plane when the frictional resistance to its motion is

    A. ignored
    B. increased slightly
    C. equal to the force pulling it down the plane
    D. slightly greater than the force pulling it down the plane

16. The differential gears on the rear axle of an automobile

    A. shift when the automatic transmission shifts
    B. enable the driver to obtain maximum speeds with minimum consumption of gasoline
    C. make it possible to use one non-skid chain effectively instead of two
    D. permit one wheel to travel faster than the other on curves

17. The laser is a device which produces light amplification through stimulated   17.____

    A. electrical reactance   B. induced magnetism
    C. emission radiation   D. frequency modulation

18. Nearsightedness is GENERALLY corrected by using a   18.____

    A. converging lens
    B. convex lens
    C. concave lens
    D. lens of focal length 13 mm.

19. If there are 4 supporting strands in the pulley system, a 400 lb. safe can be lifted (neglecting friction) by applying a force of _____ lbs.   19.____

    A. 32   B. 40   C. 100   D. 400

20. When currents are set up in a liquid through unequal heating, the heat is transferred PRINCIPALLY by   20.____

    A. conduction   B. radiation
    C. vapor pressure   D. convection

21. Which one of the following is NOT a recommended soil erosion control measure?   21.____

    A. Terracing
    B. Crop rotation
    C. Strip cropping
    D. Plowing instead of burning stubble

22. Which one of the following statements is TRUE of contour maps?   22.____

    A. The closer the contour lines, the steeper the grade.
    B. The more separated the contour lines, the steeper the grade.
    C. When contour lines become too close to distinguish, a smaller contour interval is used.
    D. Contour lines represent relief better than hachures do.

23. A very meandering course, flat topography with no falls or rapids, poor drainage on the flood plain, swampy vegetation and few tributaries are characteristic of a river in its   23.____

    A. youth   B. maturity
    C. old age   D. maturity and old age

24. Potholes, outwash plains, hanging valleys, and kames are all terms DIRECTLY associated with the activities of   24.____

    A. rivers   B. glaciers   C. volcanoes   D. mountains

25. Which one of the following statements with regard to cyclones is NOT true?   25.____

    A. Hurricanes are tropical cyclones.
    B. The air in a cyclone moves rapidly outward from the *eye*.
    C. Sooner or later, all cyclones conform to the path of the prevailing westerlies.
    D. A cyclone is merely a low pressure area and the winds within it may have any velocity.

KEY (CORRECT ANSWERS)

1.	A	11.	A
2.	D	12.	B
3.	C	13.	A
4.	D	14.	B
5.	A	15.	C
6.	B	16.	D
7.	B	17.	C
8.	C	18.	C
9.	B	19.	C
10.	C	20.	D

21. B
22. A
23. C
24. B
25. B

TEST 3

DIRECTIONS: Each question or incomplete statement is followed by several suggested answers or completions. Select the one that BEST answers the question or completes the statement. *PRINT THE LETTER OF THE CORRECT ANSWER IN THE SPACE AT THE RIGHT.*

1. The gland which produces insulin is to be found in the

    A. liver B. pituitary C. thymus D. pancreas

    1.____

2. Gamma globulins used in the protection against measles and polio contain

    A. toxoids
    C. weakened viruses
    B. dead viruses
    D. antibodies

    2.____

3. Low sodium diets are used for the

    A. prevention of edema
    B. treatment of heart disease
    C. reduction of cholesterol in the blood
    D. treatment of bacterial endocarditis

    3.____

4. Of the following diseases, the one whose causative agent is of a different type from those of the other three is

    A. diphtheria
    C. poliomyelitis
    B. tetanus
    D. typhoid fever

    4.____

5. *Do not move the patient* is a first aid precept which is applicable particularly in cases of

    A. bleeding and fainting
    C. sunstroke and asphyxia
    B. fracture and shock
    D. burns and heat exhaustion

    5.____

6. All of the following statements pertaining to items found in home medicine cabinets are correct EXCEPT:

    A. Tincture of iodine is unaffected by long storage and hence may be used indefinitely
    B. Hydrogen peroxide is usable as long as it bubbles energetically
    C. Age does not make sedatives dangerous, but they may lose some of their potency with time
    D. If the supply of bicarbonate of soda is exhausted, baking soda may be substituted

    6.____

7. Of the following, the INCORRECT association of a disease with the period of time during which it is usually communicable is

    A. impetigo - as long as the sores are unhealed
    B. measles - during the period of running eyes and nose
    C. diphtheria - usually two weeks from the onset of the infection
    D. tetanus - from the onset of the disease to one week later

    7.____

8. The group of terms which is correctly arranged in the order of increasing inclusiveness, the LEAST inclusive being stated first, is

    A. tissues, cells, systems, organs
    B. cells, organs, tissues, organisms
    C. cells, genes, organs, tissues
    D. cells, tissues, organs, systems

    8.____

9. Ascorbic acid is a vitamin whose presence in foods prevents the occurrence of

   A. beriberi
   B. night blindness
   C. scurvy
   D. rickets

10. Vitamin A deficiency is associated with all of the following EXCEPT

    A. faulty development of the teeth
    B. impairment of vision in dim light
    C. unhealthy condition of the skin and mucous membranes
    D. retardation of the development of bones

11. Aureomycin was developed by

    A. Fleming   B. Banting   C. Waksman   D. Duggar

12. A class of engines that are NOT of the internal combustion type is _____ engines.

    A. diesel
    B. gasoline
    C. turbo-jet
    D. steam

13. The lead storage battery commonly used in American auto-mobiles is filled with a solution of _____ acid.

    A. sulfuric
    B. nitric
    C. phosphoric
    D. hydrochloric

14. All stars visible to the naked eye belong to

    A. the solar system
    B. a number of galaxies
    C. the Milky Way galaxy
    D. the Milky Way galaxy and several spiral nebulae

15. A poisonous snake native to the eastern United States is the

    A. puff adder
    B. king snake
    C. milk snake
    D. water moccasin

16. When an observer hears thunder 10 seconds after he sees the lightning flash that caused it, the distance between him and the point of origin of the flash is APPROXIMATELY _____ mile(s).

    A. 1   B. 2   C. 5   D. 10

17. Rivers flowing into a lake may eventually destroy it by

    A. erosion
    B. stream piracy
    C. deposition
    D. solution

18. The metal used for the filament of the modern incandescent lamp is

    A. tungsten   B. tantalum   C. thorium   D. titanium

19. The APPROXIMATE number of miles per degree of latitude of the earth is

    A. 90   B. 70   C. 15
    D. widely variable, depending on location

20. The bedrock of a large part of Manhattan is the rock called 20._____
    A. granite   B. quartzite   C. schist   D. trap

21. The function of the cadmium rods in a nuclear reactor is to _____ neutrons. 21._____
    A. slow down   B. absorb   C. speed up   D. create

22. The BRIGHTEST star visible in the nightime sky in New York City is 22._____
    A. Betelgeuse   B. Orion   C. Polaris   D. Sirius

23. A dry cleaning fluid which is NOT flammable is 23._____
    A. carbon disulfide   B. carbon tetrachloride
    C. dimethyl phthalate   D. freon

24. The dark gray clouds that form a complete overcast on rainy days are called 24._____
    A. alto-stratus   B. nimbo-stratus
    C. cumulus   D. cirrus

25. Most of the United States lies in the terrestrial wind belt affected by the prevailing 25._____
    A. southwesterlies   B. northwesterlies
    C. southeasterlies   D. northeasterlies

KEY (CORRECT ANSWERS)

1. D		11. D	
2. D		12. D	
3. A		13. A	
4. C		14. C	
5. B		15. D	
6. A		16. B	
7. D		17. C	
8. D		18. A	
9. C		19. B	
10. D		20. D	

21. B
22. D
23. B
24. B
25. A

TEST 4

DIRECTIONS: Each question or incomplete statement is followed by several suggested answers or completions. Select the one that BEST answers the question or completes the statement. *PRINT THE LETTER OF THE CORRECT ANSWER IN THE SPACE AT THE RIGHT.*

1. In general, as latitude increases from 0° to about 30°, precipitation 1._____

    A. remains uniform
    B. increases
    C. decreases
    D. shows no particular trend

2. Heavy dew is MOST likely to form on a _____ night. 2._____

    A. calm, clear
    B. clear, windy
    C. calm, cloudy
    D. windy, overcast

3. The Catskill Mountains of New York State can BEST be described as 3._____

    A. coastal plain
    B. folded mountain
    C. plateau
    D. a series of domes

4. Bays like San Francisco Bay, Chesapeake Bay, and Delaware Bay are 4._____

    A. parts of deltas
    B. fiords
    C. artificial harbors
    D. submerged river valleys

5. When first aid is to be administered to a pupil who has been injured in the classroom, of the four measures indicated below, the one which should be given PRECEDENCE is 5._____

    A. controlling the bleeding
    B. moving the student out of the classroom
    C. sending for a doctor
    D. treating for shock

6. The normal number of teeth in the adult human being is 6._____

    A. 28   B. 32   C. 36   D. 30

7. The reproductive organs of a flowering plant are the 7._____

    A. stomata and guard cells
    B. fibrovascular bundles and sieve tubes
    C. pistils and stamens
    D. cambium layer and lenticels

8. A virus is the causative agent of 8._____

    A. malaria
    B. tetanus
    C. smallpox
    D. typhoid fever

9. In a blast furnace, the slag 9._____

    A. is drained off from below the molten iron
    B. floats on top of the molten iron
    C. is mixed with the iron to produce steel
    D. mixes with the iron when the *pigs* form

10. If iron filings are sprinkled on a sheet of paper under which the north poles of two bar magnets face one another at a distance of one and a quarter inches, the lines of force show

    A. repulsion
    B. attraction
    C. partial attraction
    D. irregularities indicating both attraction and repulsion

11. Of the following, the substance which is NOT an antibiotic is

    A. aureomycin   B. penicillin
    C. streptomycin   D. sulphanilamide

12. The electric meter in the home measures

    A. kilowatts   B. kilowatt-hours
    C. watts   D. watt-hours

13. The blood group which is COMMONLY referred to as the *universal donor* is

    A. A   B. B   C. AB   D. O

14. Renewal of the supply of oxygen in our atmosphere is accomplished CHIEFLY by the

    A. burning of wood and coal that occurs throughout the world
    B. natural decomposition of oxides found in the earth's surface
    C. photosynthetic process in plants
    D. normal loss of dissolved gases from the oceans

15. Mumps is an infection of the

    A. cervical lymph glands   B. parotid glands
    C. thyroid glands   D. tonsils

16. Radioactive iodine is used effectively in the treatment of cancer of the

    A. adrenals   B. liver   C. thymus   D. thyroid

17. In television broadcasting, light waves from the subject are changed into electrical impulses by a

    A. converter   B. detector tube
    C. photoelectric cell D. scanning disc

18. The star Polaris is found in the constellation

    A. Arcturus   B. Big Dipper
    C. Cassiopeia   D. Little Dipper

19. MOST digested food is absorbed into the bloodstream through the walls of the

    A. large intestine   B. pancreas
    C. small intestine   D. stomach

20. To test the strength of the charge of a storage battery, it is BEST to use a(n)

    A. ammeter   B. hydrometer
    C. neon test lamp   D. voltmeter

21. A body in motion remains in motion in a straight line at the same rate unless it is acted on by an external disturbing force.
    This is, in part, a statement of the law of

    A. inertia
    B. falling bodies
    C. relativity
    D. mass action

    21._____

22. Summer thunderstorms in the northeastern part of the United States are USUALLY associated with _____ clouds.

    A. cirrus B. cumulus C. nimbus D. stratus

    22._____

23. A plant grower produces a new kind of rose. He can propagate and perpetuate the new rose by

    A. cross-pollination
    B. grafting
    C. inbreeding
    D. self-pollination

    23._____

24. A catalyst

    A. alters the rate of chemical change
    B. emulsifies fats
    C. fixes a dye in fabric
    D. is a reducing agent

    24._____

25. A plant whose seeds are dispersed by the wind is the

    A. burdock
    B. coconut
    C. horse chestnut
    D. maple

    25._____

KEY (CORRECT ANSWERS)

1. C		11. D	
2. A		12. B	
3. C		13. D	
4. D		14. C	
5. A		15. B	
6. B		16. D	
7. C		17. C	
8. C		18. D	
9. B		19. C	
10. A		20. B	

21. A
22. B
23. B
24. A
25. D

TEST 5

DIRECTIONS: Each question or incomplete statement is followed by several suggested answers or completions. Select the one that BEST answers the question or completes the statement. *PRINT THE LETTER OF THE CORRECT ANSWER IN THE SPACE AT THE RIGHT.*

1. Glass is etched by a solution of _____ acid. 1._____
   - A. hydrofluoric
   - B. carbolic
   - C. nitric
   - D. sulfuric

2. The phases of the moon are caused by the 2._____
   - A. earth's revolution
   - B. earth's rotation
   - C. moon's revolution
   - D. moon's rotation

3. The Lysenko theories of inheritance have a CLOSE similarity to the theories of 3._____
   - A. De Vries
   - B. Lamarck
   - C. Mendel
   - D. Galton

4. Vitamin D is found in comparatively large amounts in 4._____
   - A. fish liver oils
   - B. citrus fruits
   - C. leafy vegetables
   - D. lean meats

5. Particularly rich uranium deposits have been found in 5._____
   - A. Belgian Congo
   - B. Iran
   - C. Mexico
   - D. Chile

6. The oceans cover _____ tenths of the surface of the earth. 6._____
   - A. three
   - B. five
   - C. seven
   - D. nine

7. The area of Europe is roughly _____ that of the United States. 7._____
   - A. half
   - B. the same as
   - C. twice
   - D. three times

8. The process LEAST likely to result in vitamin loss is 8._____
   - A. bleaching celery
   - B. refining flour
   - C. quick freezing fruits
   - D. peeling vegetables

9. The natural resource of the United States which it is commonly expected will be FIRST exhausted is 9._____
   - A. iron ore
   - B. coal
   - C. bauxite
   - D. petroleum

10. The SHORTEST distance between any two points on the earth's surface is always along a(n) 10._____
    - A. arc of a meridian
    - B. arc of a parallel of latitude
    - C. arc of a great circle
    - D. contour line

15

11. Normally, a farm in the temperate zone in order to raise most crops must have a yearly rainfall amounting to at LEAST _____ inches.

    A. 20 B. 40 C. 60 D. 80

12. A good example of a *continental climate* is found in

    A. North Dakota
    B. Florida
    C. New York
    D. Alaska

13. The word *doldrums* refers to

    A. mountains that are difficult to climb
    B. tropical islands of volcanic origin
    C. geysers that erupt irregularly
    D. parts of the ocean where calms prevail

14. At the time of the vernal equinox (about March 21st), the sun at noon is DIRECTLY over the

    A. Tropic of Capricorn and moving north
    B. Tropic of Cancer and moving south
    C. Equator and moving north
    D. Equator and moving south

15. New Year's Day will be celebrated FIRST in

    A. New York B. Rome C. Bombay D. Manila

16. Of the following sources of energy, the one which appears NOT to be exploitation of the energy radiated by the sun is

    A. coal
    B. organic food
    C. tidal power
    D. water power

17. Lime is used

    A. in blast furnaces
    B. in manufacturing cement
    C. in the production of carbonated drinks
    D. for reducing the acidity of the soil

18. An appliance in which chemical energy is changed into electrical energy is a

    A. galvanometer
    B. hydrometer
    C. storage battery
    D. thermocouple

19. Galileo noticed that black spots crossed the visible solar disc in about fourteen days. This shows that

    A. the sun rotates in about twenty-seven days
    B. the sun rotates in about fourteen days
    C. there are cyclonic storms in the sun's atmosphere somewhat like the cyclonic storms on the earth in the area of the westerlies
    D. there are volcanic craters on the sun which gradually shift their position

20. The set of prisms incorporated in a pair of field glasses 20._____

    A. changes the light path
    B. increases the illumination
    C. inverts the image
    D. reflects the image

21. Attempts have been made to improve the genetic make-up of the human race by 21._____

    A. adopting social security laws
    B. improving the food habits of large numbers of people
    C. providing better housing
    D. sterilizing the feeble-minded

22. The part of the seedless grape plant that is used in producing more seedless grape plants is the 22._____

    A. fruit   B. leaf   C. root   D. stem

23. Evergreen trees whose needles grow in clusters are 23._____

    A. balsams   B. hemlocks   C. pines   D. spruces

24. Data concerning the entire surface of the moon are NOT available because 24._____

    A. telescopes are not yet powerful enough
    B. the half of the moon which faces the earth in the daytime is not visible at night
    C. the period of rotation of the moon is exactly the same as its period of revolution
    D. until very recently radar contact with the moon had not yet been made

25. The FIRST cyclotron was devised by 25._____

    A. E.O. Lawrence
    B. Lise Meitner
    C. Robert Oppenheimer
    D. Hugh Taylor

KEY (CORRECT ANSWERS)

1. A
2. C
3. B
4. A
5. A

6. C
7. B
8. C
9. D
10. C

11. A
12. A
13. D
14. C
15. D

16. C
17. D
18. C
19. A
20. D

21. D
22. D
23. C
24. C
25. A

EXAMINATION SECTION
TEST 1

DIRECTIONS: Each question or incomplete statement is followed by several suggested answers or completions. Select the one that BEST answers the question or completes the statement. *PRINT THE LETTER OF THE CORRECT ANSWER IN THE SPACE AT THE RIGHT.*

1. The human body consists of many elements of which the one in greatest abundance is   1.____

    A. carbon   B. hydrogen   C. oxygen   D. calcium

2. Of the following foods, the one richest in fats by percentage is   2.____

    A. chocolate candy bar   B. cheddar cheese
    C. cream   D. vanilla ice cream

3. The unit of electrical energy is called the   3.____

    A. ampere   B. volt
    C. ohm   D. watt-hour

4. A diesel engine differs from a gasoline engine because it has no   4.____

    A. cylinders   B. fuel
    C. carburetor   D. manifold

5. The renowned experiments of Beadle and Tatum on the mold, Neurospora, demonstrated the   5.____

    A. fundamental relationship between genes and enzymes
    B. induction of immunity to tissue transplants
    C. role of DNA in the hereditary process
    D. unacceptability of Lysenko's theories

6. The scientist whose experiments led to the development of the barometer was   6.____

    A. Newton   B. Torricelli
    C. Oersted   D. Kepler

7. Of the following, the vitamin which the body is LEAST able to store is   7.____

    A. ascorbic acid   B. calciferol
    C. niacin   D. thiamin

8. Magdeburg hemispheres demonstrate that   8.____

    A. water exerts pressure
    B. air exerts pressure
    C. the earth is an oblate spheroid
    D. wind velocity can be measured

9. A law pertaining to pressure on gases was developed by   9.____

    A. Kelvin   B. Adams   C. Boyle   D. Banks

10. The fuel which produces the greatest amount of heat energy per pound is   10.____

    A. gasoline   B. natural gas
    C. fuel oil   D. anthracite coal

11. Molecules of steam differ from those of ice in that the molecules of steam   11.____

    A. move more slowly   B. contain less energy
    C. are closer together   D. are farther apart

12. Tannic acid is used for   12.____

    A. making paper   B. curing hides
    C. dyeing cloth   D. mixing paints

13. Submerged submarines can be located by   13.____

    A. millebars   B. radar   C. sonar   D. HF/DF

14. An instrument which indicates the number of revolutions per minute of an airplane engine is called a(n)   14.____

    A. tachometer   B. psychrometer
    C. anemometer   D. pyrometer

15. When black, rough-coated guinea pigs, hybrid for both color and texture of coat are crossed, some of their offspring are white, smooth-coated guinea pigs. This is a classic illustration of the law of   15.____

    A. independent assortment   B. dominance
    C. linkage   D. segregation

16. Which one of the following receptors is INCORRECTLY paired with the structure in which it is found?   16.____

    A. Taste bud - tongue
    B. Rod - retina
    C. Cone - retina
    D. Proprioceptor - nasal epithelium

17. A gland which acts both as a duct gland as well as a ductless gland is the   17.____

    A. thyroid   B. adrenal
    C. parathyroid   D. pancreas

18. A vitamin formerly thought to be a single compound but now known to be a complex of at least ten separate vitamins is vitamin   18.____

    A. A   B. B   C. C   D. D

19. Of the following nutrients, the one which is absorbed by the lymph, rather than by the blood in the capillaries, is   19.____

    A. amino acids   B. fatty acids
    C. glucose   D. water

20. A person of type AB blood should be given a transfusion   20.____

    A. only from O and AB
    B. only from AB and A
    C. only from AB and B
    D. from either O, A, B, or AB

21. A classic study on human gastric digestion was performed by   21.____

    A. Beaumont   B. Schleiden
    C. Pavlov   D. Banting

22. The nervous system is derived from   22.____

    A. ectoderm
    B. mesoderm
    C. endoderm
    D. a combination of endoderm and ectoderm

23. Which one of the following series is in the correct sequence?   23.____

    A. Fertilized egg, cleavage, blastula, gastrula
    B. Blastula, fertilized egg, gastrula, cleavage
    C. Blastula, cleavage, gastrula, fertilized egg
    D. Fertilized egg, blastula, cleavage, gastrula

24. Which one of the following statements regarding plant hormones is NOT true?   24.____

    A. Despite much research, auxins have thus far not been synthesized.
    B. The auxins from an oat coleoptile can be absorbed on a block of agar and used for further experimentation.
    C. Auxins accelerate lengthwise growth in the stem.
    D. Auxins retard lengthwise growth in the root.

25. In a woody stem, all growth results from the activity of the   25.____

    A. cambium   B. phloem
    C. pith   D. xylem

KEY (CORRECT ANSWERS)

1.	C	11.	D
2.	A	12.	B
3.	D	13.	C
4.	C	14.	A
5.	A	15.	A
6.	B	16.	D
7.	A	17.	D
8.	B	18.	B
9.	C	19.	B
10.	A	20.	D

21. A
22. A
23. A
24. A
25. A

TEST 2

DIRECTIONS: Each question or incomplete statement is followed by several suggested answers or completions. Select the one that BEST answers the question or completes the statement. *PRINT THE LETTER OF THE CORRECT ANSWER IN THE SPACE AT THE RIGHT.*

1. Of the following, the compound which is NOT easily combustible is   1.____

    A. CH_4 B. C_2H_2 C. CO D. CO_2

2. Chemical activity is due PRINCIPALLY to   2.____

    A. neutrons B. electrons
    C. protons   D. nucleons

3. The isotopes of an atom differ from each other in their   3.____

    A. chemical properties B. atomic mass
    C. nuclear charge   D. number of protons

4. The world's FIRST nuclear desalinization plant was constructed at which one of the following locations?   4.____

    A. Guantanamo, Cuba B. Indian Point, N.Y.
    C. Riverhead, L.I.   D. Hanford, Wash.

5. Of the following, the example of a purely physical change is   5.____

    A. fractional distillation of petroleum
    B. destructive distillation of wood
    C. cracking of petroleum products
    D. hydrogenation of cottonseed oil

6. Salt becomes ineffective in melting ice on a sidewalk when the ground temperature falls below   6.____

    A. 30° F B. 20° F C. 10° F D. 0° F

7. Of the following, the one in which sight and photography are MOST different is   7.____

    A. projecting an inverted image upon a light-sensitive surface
    B. controlling the amount of admitted light
    C. the process of focusing
    D. being able to use light-sensitive structures that differ in degree of sensitivity

8. Of the following, the one which is the MOST complete statement of the modern concept of light is that it is   8.____

    A. a steady stream of particles shot off by a luminous body
    B. a type of wave motion through space
    C. a pulsating shower of small particles of energy
    D. continuous emission and absorption of radiation

9. The bright bands of color seen when sunlight falls on a soap bubble are caused by

   A. dispersion
   B. interference
   C. pigments in the soap
   D. refraction

10. Of the following substances, the one which is NOT a good conductor of electricity is

    A. carbon
    B. sea water
    C. aluminum
    D. distilled water

11. To prevent skidding during a turn, a pilot coordinates his use of the rudder with use of which one of the following parts of an airplane?

    A. Elevators
    B. Stabilizer
    C. Flaps
    D. Ailerons

12. Of the following possible effects of specific vitamin deficiency, the one which is INCORRECT is that

    A. lack of vitamin A causes night blindness
    B. lack of vitamin K causes failure of blood clotting
    C. lack of riboflavin causes growth failure
    D. lack of vitamin B12 causes pellagra

13. The swelling of the salivary gland is a MAJOR symptom of which one of the following?

    A. Measles
    B. Chicken pox
    C. Mumps
    D. Typhoid fever

14. Teachers are expected to administer to pupils, if necessary, each of the following types of first aid EXCEPT

    A. use of pressure points to control bleeding
    B. mouth-to-mouth artificial respiration
    C. clearing the mouth of obstructions to breathing
    D. use of antiseptics on a skin wound

15. A child with ringworm of the scalp

    A. may continue to attend regular class provided he is under treatment
    B. must be excluded from school even if he is under treatment
    C. must be isolated from other children in class even if he is under treatment
    D. may remain in school even if he is not under treatment

16. A disease of children often resulting from an acute disorder and characterized principally by irregular, involuntary, and uncontrollable movements in the face or extremities is called

    A. cerebral palsy
    B. shingles
    C. chorea
    D. epilepsy

17. BCG vaccine is used to prevent

    A. measles
    B. tuberculosis
    C. whooping cough
    D. yellow fever

18. The wholesome emotional development of a child is generally MOST dependent upon which one of the following?

   A. Meaningful play equipment available to him
   B. His intelligence
   C. Attitudes of adults with whom he intimately associates
   D. Number of his siblings

18._____

19. The stadiometer is used to measure

   A. hearing   B. height   C. sight   D. weight

19._____

20. To diminish the flow of blood to the upper arm, pressure should be placed on the

   A. femoral artery   B. brachial artery
   C. carotid artery   D. pulmonary artery

20._____

21. The daily changes in tides are caused by the

   A. rotation of the earth on its axis
   B. gravitational pull of the moon
   C. gravitational pull of the sun
   D. inclination of the earth's axis

21._____

22. Alternating current can be changed into direct current through the use of a(n)

   A. transformer   B. variable resistor
   C. A.C. filter   D. rectifier

22._____

23. The gland which is generally considered to function as an endocrinological switchboard is the

   A. thyroid   B. adrenal
   C. pituitary   D. pineal

23._____

24. A claw-hammer and a pair of scissors are examples of simple machines known as

   A. pulleys   B. axles   C. wedges   D. levers

24._____

25. In order to explain Archimedes' Principle, reference should be made to the relation between the

   A. size of an object to its volume
   B. weight of an object in air and its weight in a vacuum
   C. loss of weight of an object in water and the weight of the water it displaces
   D. volume of an object and the volume of water it displaces

25._____

KEY (CORRECT ANSWERS)

1. D
2. B
3. B
4. C
5. A

6. D
7. C
8. C
9. B
10. D

11. A
12. D
13. C
14. D
15. A

16. C
17. B
18. C
19. B
20. B

21. B
22. D
23. C
24. D
25. C

TEST 3

DIRECTIONS: Each question or incomplete statement is followed by several suggested answers or completions. Select the one that BEST answers the question or completes the statement. *PRINT THE LETTER OF THE CORRECT ANSWER IN THE SPACE AT THE RIGHT.*

1. In a blast furnace, the slag

    A. is drained off from below the molten iron
    B. floats on top of the molten iron
    C. is mixed with the iron to produce steel
    D. mixes with the iron when the "pigs" form

    1.____

2. If iron filings are sprinkled on a sheet of paper under which the north poles of two bar magnets face one another at a distance of one and a quarter inches, the lines of force show

    A. repulsion
    B. attraction
    C. partial attraction
    D. irregularities indicating both attraction and repulsion

    2.____

3. Of the following, the substance which is NOT an antibiotic is

    A. aureomycin   B. penicillin
    C. streptomycin   D. sulphanilamide

    3.____

4. The electric meter in the home measures

    A. kilowatts   B. kilowatt-hours
    C. watts   D. watt-hours

    4.____

5. The blood group which is commonly referred to as the "universal donor" is

    A. A   B. B   C. AB   D. O

    5.____

6. Renewal of the supply of oxygen in our atmosphere is accomplished chiefly by the

    A. burning of wood and coal that occurs throughout the world
    B. natural decomposition of oxides found in the earth's surface
    C. photosynthetic process in plants
    D. normal loss of dissolved gases from the oceans

    6.____

7. Mumps is an infection of the

    A. cervical lymph glands   B. parotid glands
    C. thyroid glands   D. tonsils

    7.____

8. Radioactive iodine is used effectively in the treatment of cancer of the

    A. adrenals   B. liver   C. thymus   D. thyroid

    8.____

9. In television broadcasting, light waves from the subject are changed into electrical impulses by a

    A. converter   B. detector tube
    C. photoelectric cell   D. scanning disc

    9.____

10. The star Polaris is found in the constellation 10.____

    A. Arcturus B. Big Dipper
    C. Cassiopeia D. Little Dipper

11. Most digested food is absorbed into the bloodstream through the walls of the 11.____

    A. large intestine B. pancreas
    C. small intestine D. stomach

12. To test the strength of the charge of a storage battery, it is BEST to use a(n) 12.____

    A. ammeter B. hydrometer
    C. neon test lamp D. voltmeter

13. A body in motion remains in motion in a straight line at the same rate unless it is acted on 13.____
    by an external disturbing force. This is in part a statement of the law of

    A. inertia B. falling bodies
    C. relativity D. mass action

14. Summer thunderstorms in the northeastern part of the United States are usually associ- 14.____
    ated with

    A. cirrus clouds B. cumulus clouds
    C. nimbus clouds D. stratus clouds

15. When the resistance of an electrical circuit is halved and the applied voltage is doubled, 15.____
    the current in the circuit would

    A. be quadrupled B. be doubled
    C. be halved D. remain the same

16. The gyrocompass points to the 16.____

    A. prime meridian
    B. magnetic north pole
    C. geographical north pole
    D. international dateline

17. All of the following planets rotate on their axis EXCEPT 17.____

    A. Mercury B. Venus C. Earth D. Mars

18. In a second-class lever, the weight is 18.____

    A. between the fulcrum and the force
    B. separated from the force by the fulcrum
    C. separated from the fulcrum by the force
    D. is at the same point as the force

19. All of the following structures are characterized by a rich blood supply, thin membrane, 19.____
    and large surface area EXCEPT

    A. alveolus B. Bowman's capsule
    C. thrombus D. villus

20. Weather in the United States usually travels from

   A. east to west
   B. west to east
   C. north to south
   D. south to north

21. Rock that has melted and then hardened into crystals is

   A. metamorphic
   B. sedimentary
   C. glacial
   D. igneous

22. The principle of the compound bar is utilized in the

   A. thermostat
   B. aneroid barometer
   C. wind vane
   D. anemometer

23. A freely falling object falls 64 feet in

   A. 1 second
   B. 2 seconds
   C. 3 seconds
   D. 4 seconds

24. Blood carrying the highest percentage of oxygen would be found in the

   A. aorta
   B. pulmonary artery
   C. pulmonary vein
   D. vena cava

25. Ursa Major is commonly known as

   A. the swan
   B. Pegasus
   C. Cancer
   D. the Big Dipper

KEY (CORRECT ANSWERS)

1.	B	11.	C
2.	A	12.	B
3.	D	13.	A
4.	B	14.	B
5.	D	15.	A
6.	C	16.	C
7.	B	17.	B
8.	D	18.	A
9.	C	19.	C
10.	D	20.	B

21. D
22. A
23. B
24. C
25. D

TEST 4

DIRECTIONS: Each question or incomplete statement is followed by several suggested answers or completions. Select the one that BEST answers the question or completes the Statement. *PRINT THE LETTER OF THE CORRECT ANSWER IN THE SPACE AT THE RIGHT.*

1. A cathode tube is NOT used in

    A. radio
    C. amplification
    B. medicine
    D. television

    1.____

2. The planet nearest the Earth is

    A. Mars B. Jupiter C. Venus D. the moon

    2.____

3. Wind velocity is measured by a(n)

    A. weather vane
    C. baragraph
    B. anemometer
    D. hygrometer

    3.____

4. In flying from New York to Denver, you would set your watch

    A. back two hours
    C. back three hours
    B. ahead two hours
    D. ahead one hour

    4.____

5. Milk is a(n)

    A. solution
    C. compound
    B. mixture
    D. emulsion

    5.____

6. The flame of a bunsen burner strikes back when

    A. it has too much air
    B. the flame is too small
    C. it is being fed too much gas
    D. the flame is too hot

    6.____

7. When diluting a concentrated acid,

    A. pour the acid slowly into the water
    B. pour the water slowly into the acid
    C. pour acid and water simultaneously into the mixing beaker
    D. pour the water quickly into the acid

    7.____

8. For heating alcohol in a beaker in the laboratory, use

    A. a low flame
    C. live steam
    B. an alcohol burner
    D. a water bath

    8.____

9. When a fuel burns completely in air, one product that results is

    A. soot
    C. carbon monoxide
    B. carbon dioxide
    D. nitrogen

    9.____

10. Rayon is made from

    A. cellulose
    C. flax
    B. coal tar
    D. casein

    10.____

11. Exhaled air contains carbon dioxide. This can be demonstrated by   11.____

    A. using lime water
    B. using litmus paper
    C. the odor
    D. breathing on a pane of glass

12. Dry ice is   12.____

    A. solidified air
    B. supercooled water
    C. solidified ethylene chloride
    D. solidified carbon dioxide

13. A stream of hydrogen burns in the air. As a result, we get   13.____

    A. acetylene   B. hydrogen peroxide
    C. water   D. carbon dioxide

14. A dynamo converts   14.____

    A. mechanical energy into electrical energy
    B. potential energy into kinetic energy
    C. heat energy into electrical energy
    D. electrical energy into stored energy

15. A man weighing 150 pounds walks up a flight of 18 steps, each 6 inches high. In doing   15.____
    so, he does work equal in foot-pounds to

    A. 1350   B. 2750   C. 1025   D. 1800

16. You wind copper wire several times around an iron nail. The ends of the wire are   16.____
    attached to the poles of a battery. This experiment is used to demonstrate

    A. conduction   B. a rheostat
    C. induction   D. electrical resistance

17. Of the following compounds, the one readily soluble in water is   17.____

    A. calcium carbonate   B. sodium chloride
    C. aluminum oxide   D. iron oxide

18. The planet having the greatest number of known satellites is   18.____

    A. Saturn   B. Uranus   C. Mars   D. Jupiter

19. A reagent commonly used to test food for the presence of certain sugars is   19.____

    A. Lugol's   B. Dakin's
    C. Fehling's   D. Farrell's solution

20. In the summertime, moisture collects on the outside of a glass of ice water through the   20.____
    process of

    A. deliquescence   B. osmosis
    C. capillary action   D. condensation

21. When a dry cloth that has been saturated with cobalt chloride is exposed to moist air, it turns

    A. red   B. blue   C. green   D. brown

22. Carbohydrates are stored in the liver in the form of

    A. peptones   B. bile   C. glycogen   D. glucose

23. Concave glasses are used to correct

    A. ophthalmia
    C. hypermetropia
    B. strabismus
    D. myopia

24. A body, when entirely surrounded by fluid, is buoyed up by a force equal to the weight of the fluid it displaces.
    This principle is known as that of

    A. Archimedes
    C. Hippocrates
    B. Pascal
    D. Descartes

25. In man, pancreatic juice contributes to digestion in the

    A. small intestine
    C. colon
    B. stomach
    D. pancreas

KEY (CORRECT ANSWERS)

1. C
2. C
3. B
4. A
5. D

6. A
7. A
8. D
9. B
10. A

11. A
12. D
13. C
14. A
15. A

16. C
17. B
18. D
19. C
20. D

21. B
22. C
23. D
24. A
25. A

EXAMINATION SECTION
TEST 1

DIRECTIONS: Each question or incomplete statement is followed by several suggested answers or completions. Select the one that BEST answers the question or completes the statement. *PRINT THE LETTER OF THE CORRECT ANSWER IN THE SPACE AT THE RIGHT.*

1. Dry ice is

    A. solid carbon dioxide
    B. supercooled water
    C. dehydrated ice
    D. solid air

    1.____

2. Current concern with population problems has revived interest in the theories of

    A. Darwin   B. DeVries   C. Lamarck   D. Malthus

    2.____

3. A piece of wood with a specific gravity of 1.1 will

    A. sink
    B. float at the surface
    C. float with 0.1 of its volume above water
    D. float with 0.99 of its volume submerged

    3.____

4. Isotopes of elements have the same

    A. atomic weight
    B. external system of electrons
    C. number of neutrons in the nucleus
    D. number of electrons and neutrons in the nucleus

    4.____

5. Sound vibrations are transmitted most rapidly by

    A. steel   B. water   C. air   D. vacuum

    5.____

6. Graphite and diamond are allotropic forms of

    A. boron   B. cadmium   C. calcium   D. carbon

    6.____

7. The image on a kineoscope of a television set is formed by a moving beam of light. We see it as a whole picture and as a moving picture because

    A. images persist on the retina
    B. electrons make a fluorescent screen glow
    C. radiant energy stimulates the retina
    D. electrical energy is changed into light energy

    7.____

8. A large crater discovered in northern Canada not long ago was produced, most likely, by the

    A. explosion of a bomb
    B. eruption of a subterranean volcano
    C. pot-hole erosion of a glacier
    D. impact of a meteorite

    8.____

9. The fuel best adapted for present day jet airplanes is 9._____

   A. naphtha B. gasoline
   C. kerosene D. benzol

10. Which pair is INCORRECTLY matched? 10._____

    A. Brass - compound
    B. Sea water - solution
    C. Air - mixture
    D. Milk - emulsion

11. If we compare the eye with a camera, the INCORRECTLY matched pair is 11._____

    A. retina - film B. cornea - lens
    C. eyelid - lens cap D. iris - diaphragm

12. Which one of these is NOT a member of the vitamin B complex? 12._____

    A. Niacin B. Thiamin C. Lecithin D. Riboflavin

13. A theory to account for the enormous output of solar heat assumes the source to be 13._____

    A. the splitting of hydrogen atoms
    B. the destruction of matter during the synthesis of helium
    C. the breakdown of uranium to barium and krypton
    D. loss of neutrons from the sun's interior

14. A metal about to be produced in quantity to aid in the building of jet engines is 14._____

    A. gallium B. osmium C. cesium D. titanium

15. Scientists have learned the chemical elements in the sun through the use of the 15._____

    A. colorimeter B. spectroscope
    C. telescope D. thermocouple

16. $E = mc^2$. This formula expresses a relationship between energy, mass, and light. It was formulated by 16._____

    A. Michaelson B. Bohr
    C. Planck D. Einstein

17. The BEST way to rid a lawn of broadleaf weeds is to 17._____

    A. cut the grass very close to the ground
    B. spray with 2, 4-D
    C. inject DDT into the soil
    D. remove each weed individually with a hand spade

18. Glass wool is a good insulator primarily because it 18._____

    A. is light in weight
    B. includes many air spaces
    C. is non-inflammable
    D. is relatively inexpensive

19. The term COLD FRONT on a weather map refers to　　　　　　　　　　　　　　　　19.____

   A. the region included by isotherms
   B. a region having frosts
   C. an advancing mass of cold air
   D. a region where storms originate

20. Atomic reactors are located on streams. This is necessary in order to　　　　　20.____

   A. dispose easily of waste products
   B. cool the reactor
   C. facilitate the transportation of needed materials
   D. absorb the radiations in water

21. When a weather report notes nimbus clouds, we may expect　　　　　　　　　　21.____

   A. clear weather　　　　　　　　　　B. cold
   C. high winds　　　　　　　　　　　　D. rain

22. A pigeon whose cerebellum has been removed cannot　　　　　　　　　　　　22.____

   A. breathe　　　　　　　　　　　　　B. swallow food
   C. coordinate its movements　　　　D. see its food

23. The yield of gasoline from crude petroleum is increased by　　　　　　　　　　23.____

   A. cracking and hydrogenation
   B. distillation and cracking
   C. distillation and emulsification
   D. hydrogenation and emulsification

24. An effective aid in curing pernicious anemia is　　　　　　　　　　　　　　　　24.____

   A. niacin　　　　　　　　　　　　　　B. histamine
   C. chloromycetin　　　　　　　　　　D. vitamin B12

25. An electric iron on a 110 volt circuit uses 6 amperes of current. How many kilowatt hours　25.____
    of electricity would it use in 5 hours of ironing?

   A. 33　　　　B. 3.3　　　　C. 330　　　　D. 3300

KEY (CORRECT ANSWERS)

1.	A	11.	B
2.	D	12.	C
3.	A	13.	B
4.	B	14.	D
5.	A	15.	B
6.	D	16.	D
7.	A	17.	B
8.	D	18.	B
9.	C	19.	C
10.	A	20.	B

21. D
22. C
23. A
24. D
25. B

TEST 2

DIRECTIONS: Each question or incomplete statement is followed by several suggested answers or completions. Select the one that BEST answers the question or completes the statement. *PRINT THE LETTER OF THE CORRECT ANSWER IN THE SPACE AT THE RIGHT.*

1. Of the following diseases, the one whose causative agent is of a different type from those of the other three is

    A. diphtheria
    B. tetanus
    C. poliomyelitis
    D. typhoid fever

    1.____

2. "Do not move the patient" is a first-aid precept which is applicable particularly in cases of

    A. bleeding and fainting
    B. fracture and shock
    C. sunstroke and asphyxia
    D. burns and heat exhaustion

    2.____

3. All of the following statements pertaining to items found in home medicine cabinets are correct EXCEPT:

    A. Tincture of iodine is unaffected by long storage and hence may be used indefinitely
    B. Hydrogen peroxide is usable as long as it bubbles energetically
    C. Age does not make sedatives dangerous, but they may lose some of their potency with time
    D. If the supply of bicarbonate of soda is exhausted, baking soda may be substituted

    3.____

4. Of the following, the INCORRECT association of a disease with the period of time during which it is usually communicable is

    A. impetigo - as long as the sores are unhealed
    B. measles - during the period of running eyes and nose
    C. diphtheria - usually two weeks from the onset of the infection
    D. tetanus - from the onset of the disease to one week later

    4.____

5. The group of terms which is CORRECTLY arranged in the order of increasing inclusiveness, the least inclusive being stated first, is

    A. tissues, cells, systems, organs
    B. cells, organs, tissues, organisms
    C. cells, genes, organs, tissues
    D. cells, tissues, organs, systems

    5.____

6. Ascorbic acid is a vitamin whose presence in foods prevents the occurrence of

    A. beriberi
    B. night blindness
    C. scurvy
    D. rickets

    6.____

7. Vitamin A deficiency is associated with all of the following EXCEPT

    A. faulty development of the teeth
    B. impairment of vision in dim light

    7.____

C. unhealthy condition of the skin and mucous membranes
D. retardation of the development of bones

8. Aureomycin was developed by

    A. Fleming   B. Banting   C. Waksman   D. Duggar

9. The artificial earth satellites that were planned during the International Geophysical Year by the United States circled the earth in approximately

    A. 1 1/2 hours   B. 1 1/2 days
    C. 1 1/2 weeks   D. 1 1/2 months

10. A class of engines that are NOT of the internal combustion type is

    A. diesel engines   B. gasoline engines
    C. turbo-jet engines   D. steam engines

11. The lead storage battery commonly used in American automobiles is filled with a solution of

    A. sulfuric acid   B. nitric acid
    C. phosphoric acid   D. hydrochloric acid

12. All stars visible to the naked eye belong to

    A. the solar system
    B. a number of galaxies
    C. the Milky Way galaxy
    D. the Milky Way galaxy and several spiral nebulae

13. A poisonous snake native to the eastern United States is the

    A. puff adder   B. king snake
    C. milk snake   D. water moccasin

14. When an observer hears thunder 10 seconds after he sees the lightning flash that caused it, the distance between him and the point of origin of the flash is approximately

    A. 1 mile   B. 2 miles   C. 5 miles   D. 10 miles

15. Rivers flowing into a lake may eventually destroy it by

    A. erosion   B. stream piracy
    C. deposition   D. solution

16. The metal used for the filament of the modern incandescent lamp is

    A. tungsten   B. tantalum   C. thorium   D. titanium

17. The approximate number of miles per degree of latitude of the earth is

    A. 90
    B. 70
    C. 15
    D. widely variable, depending on location

18. The bedrock of a large part of Manhattan is the rock called 18.____

   A. granite B. quartzite
   C. schist   D. trap

19. The function of the cadmium rods in a nuclear reactor is to 19.____

   A. slow down neutrons   B. absorb neutrons
   C. speed up neutrons   D. create neutrons

20. The brightest star visible in the night time in New York City is 20.____

   A. Betelgeuse   B. Orion
   C. Polaris   D. Sirius

21. A dry cleaning fluid which is not flammable is 21.____

   A. carbon disulfide   B. carbon tetrachloride
   C. dimethyl phthalate   D. freon

22. The purpose of making a simple anemometer for a primary grade science lesson is to develop the concept that 22.____

   A. air takes up space
   B. the wind blows from different directions
   C. strong winds can destroy things
   D. the wind blows with different amounts of force

23. The normal number of teeth in the adult human being is 23.____

   A. 28   B. 32   C. 36   D. 30

24. The reproductive organs of a flowering plant are the 24.____

   A. stomata and guard cells
   B. fibrovascular bundles and sieve tubes
   C. pistils and stamens
   D. cambium layer and lenticles

25. A virus is the causative agent of 25.____

   A. malaria   B. tetanus
   C. smallpox   D. typhoid fever

KEY (CORRECT ANSWERS)

1. C
2. B
3. A
4. D
5. D

6. C
7. D
8. D
9. A
10. D

11. A
12. C
13. D
14. B
15. C

16. A
17. B
18. C
19. B
20. D

21. B
22. D
23. B
24. C
25. C

TEST 3

DIRECTIONS: Each question or incomplete statement is followed by several suggested answers or completions. Select the one that BEST answers the question or completes the statement. *PRINT THE LETTER OF THE CORRECT ANSWER IN THE SPACE AT THE RIGHT.*

1. Which one of the following pairs is INCORRECTLY matched? 1.____

    A. Strawberry - eyes
    B. Raspberry - layers
    C. Onion - bulbs
    D. Potato - tubers

2. It was a relatively simple task for Mendel to secure pure lines in the garden pea since in nature it is 2.____

    A. wind-pollinated
    B. insect-pollinated
    C. water-pollinated
    D. self-pollinated

3. Respiration in plants 3.____

    A. is similar to respiration in animals and takes place at all times
    B. is similar to respiration in animals and takes place only when the plant is not carrying on photosynthesis
    C. is different from respiration in animals and takes place at all times
    D. is different from respiration in animals and takes place only when the plant is not carrying on photosynthesis

4. Modern research indicates that photosynthesis consists 4.____

    A. only of rapid light reactions
    B. only of slow light reactions
    C. only of a dark reaction
    D. of a light reaction followed by a dark reaction

5. Cells obtain energy quickly through 5.____

    A. photosynthesis
    B. oxidation of glucose
    C. hydrolysis of ATP
    D. osmosis

6. Which one of the following statements with regard to enzymes is NOT true? 6.____

    A. Enzymes are organic catalysts produced by living cells.
    B. Enzymes are specific, frequently acting only upon a single substrate.
    C. An enzyme can accelerate a specific reaction in only one direction.
    D. Enzymes have a protein component.

7. A reduction division takes place 7.____

    A. only in animal cells during mitosis
    B. only in plant cells during mitosis
    C. in both plant and animal cells during mitosis
    D. in both plant and animal cells during meiosis

8. The essential determiner of heredity in every living cells is a substance known as 8.____

    A. DNA   B. ACTH   C. 2-4D   D. ATP

9. If the number of protons in the nucleus of each atom is the same as the number in every other atom, the substance is

   A. inert
   B. an active non-metal
   C. amphoteric
   D. an element

10. Of the following atomic particles, the lightest in weight is the

    A. proton
    B. electron
    C. alpha particle
    D. neutron

11. The principal difference between a mixture and a chemical compound is that a

    A. mixture is always heterogeneous in composition
    B. mixture does not contain chemical substances
    C. compound is always of definite composition
    D. compound is more easily separated into its constituent parts

12. Boiling is an effective method of purifying water that contains

    A. soluble organic impurities
    B. bacteria and dissolved gases
    C. insoluble inorganic impurities
    D. soluble organic impurities and bacteria

13. An inexpensive, readily available raw material for the chemical manufacture of washing soda, hydrochloric acid and chlorine is

    A. NaCl
    B. Na_2CO_3
    C. HCl
    D. $Na_2CO_3 10H_2O$

14. About 75% of the air by weight is

    A. carbon dioxide
    B. argon
    C. oxygen
    D. nitrogen

15. Argon gas is used to fill tungsten filament electric light bulbs because it

    A. supports the combustion of the filament
    B. offers less resistance to the flow of current than nitrogen
    C. is inert and slows the evaporation of the filament
    D. is less expensive than pure oxygen

16. The number of sub-atomic particles that have been identified is

    A. ten
    B. twenty-five
    C. fifty
    D. one hundred

17. In ordinary chemical reactions, atoms combine with each other when

    A. electrons are transferred from one atom to the other
    B. nuclear particles are shared
    C. one atom loses protons gained by the other
    D. the transfer of particles produces ions with no electrical charge

18. Adenine, thymine, cytosine, and guanine are all

   A. chemical names for common vitamins
   B. units that constitute the genetic code of DNA
   C. important hormones
   D. enzymes active in digestion

19. A gas distributed commercially in solid form for use as a refrigerant is

   A. chlorine
   B. carbon dioxide
   C. argon
   D. nitrogen

20. Paraffin wax used to make candles is obtained commercially by

   A. the cracking of kerosene
   B. the dehydrogenation of fuel oil
   C. the fractional distillation of crude oil
   D. polymerization of pure hydrocarbons

21. The E.M.F. that pushes electrons through an electrical circuit is measured in

   A. ohms   B. volts   C. coulombs   D. amperes

22. The eye abnormality called hyperopic is COMMONLY known as

   A. astigmatism
   B. farsightedness
   C. nearsightedness
   D. pink eye

23. The human body is composed MAINLY of which one of the following groups of elements?

   A. Calcium, phosphorus, iron
   B. Iodine, nitrogen, calcium
   C. Carbon, hydrogen, oxygen
   D. Potassium, oxygen, iron

24. Which one of the following vitamins is NOT a member of the vitamin "B" complex?

   A. Thiamine
   B. Ascorbic acid
   C. Folic acid
   D. Niacin

25. Studies indicate that, of the following, the MOST effective procedure for reducing air pollution in cities would be to

   A. prevent the burning of trash within city limits
   B. use devices to reduce smoke coming from smokestacks
   C. establish controls reducing the discharge of gases from industrial plants
   D. use devices reducing the toxic substances thrown off in the incompletely burned exhausts of automobiles

KEY (CORRECT ANSWERS)

1.	A	11.	C
2.	D	12.	B
3.	A	13.	A
4.	D	14.	D
5.	C	15.	C
6.	C	16.	D
7.	D	17.	A
8.	A	18.	B
9.	D	19.	B
10.	B	20.	C

21. B
22. B
23. C
24. B
25. D

TEST 4

DIRECTIONS: Each question or incomplete statement is followed by several suggested answers or completions. Select the one that BEST answers the question or completes the statement. *PRINT THE LETTER OF THE CORRECT ANSWER IN THE SPACE AT THE RIGHT.*

1. A volt is a unit which measures

    A. electrical pressure
    B. electrical resistance
    C. flow of electricity
    D. volume of electricity

    1.____

2. A room temperature of 68° F is the same as a centigrade temperature of

    A. 34° C   B. 20° C   C. 15° C   D. 42° C

    2.____

3. A calorie is a

    A. substance in food
    B. measure of temperature
    C. substance that produces fat
    D. quantity of heat

    3.____

4. The number of grams equal to one ounce is, approximately,

    A. 2   B. 28   C. 83   D. 12

    4.____

5. A bus comes to a sudden stop. Standing passengers sway forward because of

    A. imbalance
    B. inertia
    C. high center of gravity
    D. centripetal force

    5.____

6. Fanning cools one because it

    A. brings cool air to the surface of the body
    B. blows away warm air
    C. promotes evaporation of perspiration
    D. reduces humidity

    6.____

7. In demonstrating combustion in a small model gas engine, the gasoline becomes ignited. The best extinguisher, of those listed, is

    A. water
    B. an air blower
    C. sawdust
    D. a towel

    7.____

8. Glass wool is a good insulator because it

    A. will not burn
    B. is inexpensive
    C. has many air spaces
    D. is inorganic

    8.____

9. A boy tries to reach for a coin which fell into a pond. He cannot pick it up where it appears to be because of

    A. refraction
    B. reflection
    C. diffraction
    D. diffusion

    9.____

10. Spontaneous generation is an attempted explanation of

    A. the origin of species
    B. how some fires start
    C. birth
    D. origin of living from non-living matter

11. A plant pigment used in the making of starch is

    A. chlorophyl   B. carotin
    C. hemoglobin   D. aniline

12. The sunshine vitamin is

    A. ascorbic acid   B. vitamin A
    C. vitamin D   D. thiamin

13. Pasteurized milk is

    A. milk from inspected cows
    B. milk that has been boiled to kill germs
    C. milk that is free from bacteria
    D. milk that has been heated to a temperature of 145° F

14. In 1892, Newark began to purify its drinking water. This has resulted in a marked reduction in death from

    A. tuberculosis   B. infantile paralysis
    C. typhoid fever   D. malaria

15. Penicillin is a(n)

    A. germicide   B. antibiotic
    C. antiseptic   D. disinfectant

16. A disease of white corpuscles is

    A. pernicious anemia   B. leukemia
    C. malaria   D. phagocytosis

17. Sulfa drugs have been used successfully in treating

    A. cancer   B. rickets
    C. infantile paralysis D. pneumonia

18. Some animals and plants can live under water because they

    A. do not need oxygen
    B. use dissolved oxygen
    C. decompose water molecules to get oxygen
    D. use water in place of oxygen

19. Some plants can make direct use of nitrogen from the air as a result of the process of

    A. absorption   B. osmosis
    C. infiltration   D. fixation

20. A natural body defense against disease germs is 20.____

   A. fresh air
   B. saliva
   C. white corpuscles
   D. enzymes

21. Seasons result from 21.____

   A. the revolution and the rotation of the earth
   B. the revolution and the inclination of the earth
   C. the variation of the distance of the earth from the sun
   D. the variation in radiation from the sun

22. A mutant is 22.____

   A. a plant graft
   B. a dumb person
   C. a hybrid
   D. an organism with a new heritable trait

23. The Dick test is a test for susceptibility to 23.____

   A. diphtheria
   B. scarlet fever
   C. tuberculosis
   D. virus infection

24. For an average-sized man doing moderately hard physical work, the caloric intake per day should be close to 24.____

   A. 6000 calories
   B. 2000 calories
   C. 3500 calories
   D. 1200 calories

25. In a balanced diet for an average person, the proportion of carbohydrates, fats, and proteins should be 25.____

   A. 2:2:1   B. 3:2:1   C. 3:1:1   D. 1:2:1

KEY (CORRECT ANSWERS)

1.	A	11.	A
2.	B	12.	C
3.	D	13.	D
4.	B	14.	C
5.	B	15.	B
6.	C	16.	B
7.	D	17.	D
8.	C	18.	B
9.	A	19.	D
10.	D	20.	C

21. B
22. D
23. B
24. C
25. C

EXAMINATION SECTION

TEST 1

DIRECTIONS: Each question or incomplete statement is followed by several suggested answers or completions. Select the one that BEST answers the question or completes the statement. *PRINT THE LETTER OF THE CORRECT ANSWER IN THE SPACE AT THE RIGHT.*

1. The sebaceous glands are associated with all of the following EXCEPT
   A. cerumen   B. true skin   C. sweat   D. oil

2. Of the following, the one NOT found in the middle ear is the
   A. cochlea   B. malleus   C. incus   D. stapes

3. All of the following concerning the digestive tract are correct EXCEPT:
   A. The larynx is between the esophagus and the epiglottis.
   B. The duodenum is between the stomach and the jejunum.
   C. The cecum is between the ileum and the colon.
   D. The vermiform process originates from the cecum.

4. The aorta arises from the
   A. right atrium
   B. left ventricle
   C. left atrium
   D. right ventricle

5. All of the following concerning red blood cells are correct EXCEPT that they
   A. possess ameboid powers
   B. are non-nucleated
   C. originate in the red marrow of the bones
   D. are stored in the spleen

6. As a rule, hyperopia is corrected by
   A. the use of convex lenses
   B. wearing dark lenses
   C. corneal transplant
   D. the use of a concave lens

7. As a rule, the MOST common method for screening vision is by using the test for
   A. muscle balance
   B. visual acuity
   C. color blindness
   D. peripheral vision

8. Internal medication should NOT be administered to students by non-medical school personnel
   A. *except* in emergencies
   B. *except* in cases where the student is accustomed to using the medication
   C. *even* in emergencies
   D. *except* when the teacher personally gives the medication

9. The grating of the broken pieces of bone in a simple fracture is called
   A. crepitus   B. contusion   C. chorisis   D. comminution

10. All of the following associations of pressure points and bleeding points are correct EXCEPT:
    A. Brachial artery – bleeding from the wrist
    B. Carotid artery – bleeding from the shoulder joint
    C. Subclavian artery – bleeding from the arm
    D. Femoral artery – bleeding from the lower leg

11. Of the following associations of fractures and distinguishing characteristics, the CORRECT one is:
    A. Colles' fracture – radial bone
    B. Compound fracture – point of fracture in contact with the external surface of the body
    C. Pott's fracture – tibiofibular joint
    D. Greenstick fracture – broken ends of the bone are interlocked

12. When taking an oral temperature, the thermometer should remain in the mouth for at least _____ minute(s).
    A. 10   B. 3   C. 2   D. 1

13. All of the following are regulators of the vital processes in the human body EXCEPT
    A. ptyalin   B. bile   C. pyridoxine   D. throxine

14. The American Dental Association urges that, of the following, the one NOT to be given to children for between-meal snacks is
    A. soft drinks   B. popcorn   C. fresh fruit   D. nuts

15. In regard to the teeth, it is CORRECT to state that the
    A. root is surrounded by enamel
    B. exterior coat of the crown is dentine
    C. neck of the tooth is at the junction of the crown and the root
    D. pulp cavity is surrounded by cementum

16. The period of deciduous dentition lasts until the
    A. individual is three years old
    B. appearance of the first permanent molar
    C. completion of the eruption of the third molars
    D. mouth has a total of 32 teeth

17. In "screening" for participation in physical education activities, the examination which should PRECEDE all others is the
    A. posture and orthopedic examination
    B. height-weight-age coefficient
    C. medical appraisal
    D. motor ability test

18. When taking an oral temperature, one should avoid all of the following EXCEPT
    A. touching the mercury bulb
    B. having the mercury register above 96 at the start
    C. placing the mercury bulb end of the thermometer under the individual's tongue
    D. taking the temperature directly after eating or drinking

    18.____

19. The MOST common type of poor posture noted in adolescent students is
    A. scoliosis   B. lordosis
    C. kyphosis   D. dypho-lordosis

    19.____

20. The use of arch supports for flat feet aims to
    A. strengthen the muscles of the feet   B. relieve pain
    C. cure the condition   D. develop stronger arches

    20.____

21. Chronic poor posture is LEAST likely to be associated with
    A. defective hearing
    B. resumption of work after recuperation from illness
    C. depressed feelings
    D. prolonged ill-health

    21.____

22. Of the following foods, the one that does NOT contain all of the indispensable amino acids is
    A. fish   B. gelatin   C. eggs   D. meat

    22.____

23. A disease caused by a thiamine deficiency is
    A. scurvy   B. keratitis   C. polyneuritis   D. pellagro

    23.____

24. Foods which provide for growth and body repair must be rich in
    A. carbohydrates   B. fats   C. minerals   D. proteins

    24.____

25. Of the following, the one which is the BEST source of iron is
    A. milk   B. liver   C. prunes   D. cheese

    25.____

KEY (CORRECT ANSWERS)

1. C
2. A
3. A
4. B
5. A

6. A
7. B
8. C
9. A
10. B

11. D
12. B
13. B
14. A
15. C

16. B
17. C
18. C
19. C
20. B

21. B
22. B
23. C
24. D
25. B

TEST 2

DIRECTIONS: Each question or incomplete statement is followed by several suggested answers or completions. Select the one that BEST answers the question or completes the statement. *PRINT THE LETTER OF THE CORRECT ANSWER IN THE SPACE AT THE RIGHT.*

1. Of the following, the BEST source of vitamins is 1.____
 A. injections B. capsules C. tablets D. foods

2. The two elements MOST vitally concerned with the building of red blood cells are 2.____
 A. calcium and potassium B. iron and copper
 C. sodium and sulfur D. chlorine and phosphorous

3. Two minerals present in combined form in the bones and teeth are 3.____
 A. calcium and phosphorous B. iron and chlorine
 C. sodium and iron D. potassium and magnesium

4. Yeast contains all of the following EXCEPT 4.____
 A. ascorbic acid B. riboflavin C. thiamin D. niacin

5. Carotene is changed to vitamin A CHIEFLY in the 5.____
 A. liver B. pancreas
 C. small intestine D. large intestine

6. Foods which ordinarily will NOT start the process of dental decay are 6.____
 A. cakes B. carbonated beverages
 C. meats D. preserves

7. Peanut butter 7.____
 A. may be used as a replacement for butter because it contains approximately the same amount of fat
 B. may be used as a replacement for fortified oleomargarine
 C. supplies a large amount of vitamin A
 D. may be used as a supplement to butter or fortified oleomargarine because it contains less fat but more protein

8. Of the following statements, the CORRECT one is that protein 8.____
 A. is stored as glycogen
 B. releases a large quantity of energy as it is oxidized
 C. is the principal nutrient in molasses
 D. is the only nutrient which contains nitrogen

9. It is authoritatively estimated that 1,000,000 people do NOT know that they have 9.____
 A. cancer B. diabetes
 C. heart disease D. tuberculosis

10. Of the following, the disturbance that has NOT as yet been detected by x-ray is
    A. diabetes
    B. gallbladder
    C. mastoid infection
    D. nasal sinus

11. Of the following associations of term and description, the INCORRECT one is:
    A. Opthalmologist – an expert in disorders of the eye
    B. Pediatrist – a specialist in children's diseases
    C. Neurologist – an expert in diseases of the nervous system
    D. Otologist – an expert in ear, nose, and throat surgery

12. ACTH is secreted by the
    A. pituitary gland
    B. adrenal glands
    C. gonads
    D. thymus gland

13. The term "trace element" is applied to
    A. the use of patch tests to determine allergies
    B. minerals present in foods in very small amounts
    C. hereditary factors
    D. symptomatic indications of illnesses

14. The type of tuberculosis that is MOST frequent between the ages of 10 and 14 is
    A. pulmonary
    B. bovine
    C. lipoid
    D. meninges

15. Of the following, the one NOT associated with tuberculosis is
    A. Mantoux
    B. Curie
    C. Koch
    D. Trudeau

16. Of the following reasons for the exclusion of coffee from children's diets, the INCORRECT one is that
    A. there is no actual nourishment in coffee except for the cream and sugar that may be added
    B. children may be adversely affected by the stimulation provided by it
    C. it usually replaces beverages that are much more important for growth
    D. it is almost always associated with all cases of malnutrition

17. In the testing of eyesight by means of the Snellen Chart, it is recommended that
    A. each eye should be tested separately and, then, both eyes tested together
    B. if a child wears glasses, the nurse should test first without glasses, then with glasses
    C. it is not necessary to test beyond the 20-foot line on the chart
    D. a reading of a line is considered satisfactory if all of the symbols or letters in that line are read correctly

18. Of the following statements concerning the hygiene of normal skin, the INCORRECT one is that
    A. warm water and a mild soap are the best known cleansing agents
    B. soaps with a large alkaline content tend to irritate the skin
    C. soaps for the face should be different from soaps for the remainder of the body
    D. the nourishment for the skin of the face comes primarily from within rather than outside the body

19. It is INCORRECT to state that ultraviolet rays
    A. act upon the ergosterol of the skin and transform it into vitamin D
    B. in many cities are filtered out by dust and smoke in the air
    C. are less effective in higher altitudes where the air is rare and dry
    D. are more intense in the spring and summer than in the fall and winter

20. The cerebellum is the part of the brain that
    A. receives messages from the sense organs
    B. contains the association area
    C. controls the coordinations of muscular movements
    D. stores memories of past events

21. Of the following associations, the INCORRECT one is:
    A. George Dick – diphtheria   B. Joseph Lister – asepsis
    C. Alexander Fleming – penicillin   D. Paul Ehrlich – bacterial diseases

22. Preventive medicine began with the work of
    A. Banting   B. Pasteur   C. Shick   D. Salk

23. It is INCORRECT to state that
    A. approximately 90% of heart disease among children of school age is caused by rheumatic fever
    B. new attacks of rheumatic manifestations are more common in the winter and spring than in other seasons
    C. throughout childhood, there is an uninterrupted rise in the incidence of rheumatic manifestations
    D. the peak of incidence of first attacks of the rheumatic infection is between the eighth and tenth years

24. Among the more definite signs of rheumatic fever are(is)
    A. a slight fever during the day
    B. painful, inflamed joints
    C. twitching of the face, arms, or legs
    D. digestive disturbances

25. Of the following associations, the INCORRECT one is: 25._____
   A. Apnea – superfluity of oxygen
   B. Dyspnea – scarcity of oxygen
   C. Eupnea – increase in depth of respiration
   D. Asphyxia – deprivation of oxygen and an excessive accumulation of carbon dioxide

KEY (CORRECT ANSWERS)

1.	D	11.	D
2.	B	12.	A
3.	A	13.	B
4.	A	14.	A
5.	A	15.	B
6.	C	16.	D
7.	D	17.	A
8.	D	18.	C
9.	B	19.	C
10.	A	20.	C

21.	A
22.	B
23.	D
24.	B
25.	C

EXAMINATION SECTION
TEST 1

DIRECTIONS: Each question or incomplete statement is followed by several suggested answers or completions. Select the one that BEST answers the question or completes the statement. *PRINT THE LETTER OF THE CORRECT ANSWER IN THE SPACE AT THE RIGHT.*

1. All of the following are associated with movement of the femur at the hip joint EXCEPT:
   A. Flexion - outward rotation
   B. Inversion – supination
   C. Inward rotation – circumduction
   D. Extension - abduction

   1.____

2. Of the following, the one necessary for the formation of thyroxin, which controls the metabolic rate, is
   A. phosphorus
   B. sodium chloride
   C. iodine
   D. calcium

   2.____

3. Excluding the coronary circulation, the average time for the complete circulation of the blood through all the circuits of the adult human body is APPROXIMATELY
   A. 23 seconds
   B. 5 minutes
   C. 1 minute, 15 seconds
   D. 10 minutes

   3.____

4. All of the following associations are correct EXCEPT:
   A. Myocarditis – inflammation of the valves of the heart
   B. Pericarditis – inflammation of the sac enveloping the heart
   C. Endocarditis – inflammation of the lining membrane of the heart
   D. Aortitis – inflammation of the vessel leading out of the lower left chamber of the heart

   4.____

5. All of the following are directly associated with the heart beat EXCEPT the
   A. pacemaker
   B. semilunar valves
   C. right atrium
   D. bundle of His

   5.____

6. Of the following, the substance necessary for the clotting of blood is
   A. ptyalin   B. prothrombin   C. gastrin   D. rennin

   6.____

7. Of the following, the ones which CANNOT be converted into heat or other forms of energy are
   A. fats   B. proteins   C. minerals   D. carbohydrates

   7.____

8. Of the following reasons for recommending cod liver oil for growing children, the INCORRECT one is that it
   A. contains a vitamin which is a growth factor for the young
   B. aids digestion of other foods
   C. is an inexpensive source of vitamins A and D

9. Of the following suggestions for reducing weight, the one MOST likely to be given by doctors to their otherwise healthy patients is to
   A. omit all desserts and bread
   B. increase the protein intake, to omit duplication in starches at each meal, and to eat low calorie desserts
   C. omit potatoes, bread, and all desserts except fruit for the main meal
   D. follow a diet made up entirely of protein, fruit, and vegetables

10. As a rule, the one which has the LONGEST incubation period is
    A. chickenpox   B. diphtheria   C. scarlet fever   D. influenza

11. All of the following associations are correct EXCEPT:
    A. Parotid gland – mumps
    B. Adrenal gland – Addison's disease
    C. Parathyroid gland – acromegaly
    D. Pituitary gland - gigantism

12. Blood sugar is LOW
    A. in untreated diabetes mellitus
    B. during emotional stress
    C. after meals
    D. during severe and prolonged muscular exertion

13. All of the following statements are correct EXCEPT:
    A. A group of symptoms that occur together and characterize a disease is a syndrome.
    B. A turning point in a disease in which a decisive change one way or another is impending is known as the crisis.
    C. The prognosis of a disease is a prediction of the disease's duration, course, and termination.
    D. A sequela of a disease is a chronic condition of the disease that persists throughout its course.

14. Active immunity may be acquired in all of the following ways EXCEPT by
    A. injections of dead bacteria or their toxins
    B. recovery from certain diseases
    C. injections of phagocytes into the bloodstream
    D. the cumulative effect of several slight exposures to certain diseases

15. All of the following associations are correct EXCEPT:
    A. Dynamometer – measuring muscle strength
    B. Manometer – measures strength of hand grip
    C. Anthropometry – measurement of the body or its various parts
    D. Ergometer – calculates work performed by a muscle or group of muscles over a specified time

16. The substances which are NOT necessary for building new tissues are
    A. water
    B. carbohydrates
    C. proteins
    D. minerals

17. A nutrient functions in any or all of the following ways EXCEPT
    A. furnish energy
    B. provide materials for building or maintenance of body tissues
    C. help regulate body processes
    D. purify the blood

18. It is MOST important to see that reducing diets of adolescents do NOT lack
    A. fats
    B. proteins
    C. carbohydrates
    D. simple sugars

19. The CHIEF value of cellulose in the diet is that it
    A. is more soluble than starch
    B. gives bulk to the intestinal residues
    C. is easily digested
    D. provides an essential amino acid

20. It is CORRECT to state that enzymes
    A. are used up in chemical reactions of foods
    B. retard the process of breaking down of foods
    C. work only in acid surroundings
    D. are specific in their action

21. All of the following are important functions of fat EXCEPT that it
    A. supports and protects organs
    B. prevents the loss of heat from the body surface
    C. is used in the building and repairing of tissues
    D. serves as a reserve supply of fuel

22. All of the following concerning cheese made from whole milk are correct EXCEPT that it
    A. preserves its milk nutrients for longer periods than the liquid itself
    B. is readily digested provided it is eaten slowly and in moderation
    C. loses its fat value when cooked
    D. is a source of riboflavin

23. The sugar which can be used by the body without having to be broken down into simpler sugars is
    A. lactose
    B. glucose
    C. maltose
    D. sucrose

24. The cells which have the property of engulfing and digesting foreign particles harmful to the body are called
    A. osteocytes   B. phagocytes   C. mast   D. plasma

25. The INCORRECT association of covering and tissue is:
    A. Periosteum – bone
    B. Perimysium – muscle
    C. Peritoneum – heart
    D. Perichondrium - cartilage

26. An acquired reduction in size of an organ which has previously reached mature size is called
    A. hyperothrophy   B. atrophy   C. necrosis   D. calcification

27. All of the following associations are correct EXCEPT:
    A. Myocardial – pertaining to the heart muscle
    B. Myoneural – pertaining to both muscle and nerve
    C. Myogenic – having origin in the muscle
    D. Myocytic – pertaining to muscular spasm

28. All of the following are concerned with the clotting of blood EXCEPT
    A. cholesterol
    B. blood platelets
    C. vitamin K
    D. prothrombin

29. Blood plays an important role in all of the following EXCEPT in the
    A. removal of waste products
    B. regulation of body temperature
    C. maintenance of water balance
    D. production of acidity of body fluids

30. Of the following, the gland MOST closely related to muscular efficiency is the
    A. adrenal   B. gonads   C. pituitary   D. thyroid

31. The INCORRECT association of gland and location is:
    A. Pineal – brain cavity
    B. Parotid – below and in front of the ear
    C. Sumaxillary – below each lower jaw
    D. Thymus – at the larynx

32. The LARGEST source of body heat is the _____ system.
    A. digestive   B. muscular   C. tegumentary   D. nervous

33. The three points of support of the longitudinal arch of the foot include all of the following EXCEPT the
    A. anterior head of the first metatarsal bone
    B. anterior head of the fifth metatarsal bone
    C. anterior head of the astragalus
    D. calcaneus

34. Long bone growth is at its maximum in the _____ period. 34.____
   A. adolescent B. pre-adolescent
   C. early childhood D. infancy

35. The acetabulum is the articular cup in a one which acts as a socket for the 35.____
   A. clavicle B. femur C. radius D. tibia

36. Of the following associations, the CORRECT one is: 36.____
   A. Second class lever – the forearm when it is being extended by the triceps muscle
   B. Third class lever – the foot when rising on the toes
   C. First class lever – the head tipping forward and backward
   D. Second class lever – the arm when it is raised sideward-upward by the deltoid muscle

37. The INCORRECT statement is: 37.____
   A. The heart of the adolescent is especially vulnerable to the stress of exercise.
   B. Exercise tolerance of children is usually higher than that of adults.
   C. Cardiac examinations have shown that the world's best athletic performers in the Olympics have hearts larger than normal.
   D. Participation in competitive athletics should be postponed pending complete recovery after infections.

38. Blood pressure is associated with all of the following EXCEPT the 38.____
   A. force of the heart beat
   B. elasticity of the walls of the blood vessels
   C. number of leucocytes present in the blood
   D. viscosity of the blood

39. In infancy _____ is(are) more rapid than in adulthood. 39.____
   A. the heart beat B. the oxidation processes
   C. the respiration rate D. all of the above

40. All of the following are correct principles relating to the muscular system EXCEPT: 40.____
   A. Muscles contract more rapidly following warm-up activities.
   B. Muscular strength is progressively developed by the repetition of exercises of the same intensity.
   C. Muscles contract more forcefully if they are first stretched, provided that they are not overstretched.
   D. A muscle must be loaded beyond its customary load if strength is to be increased.

41. Gradations in muscular contraction are related to 41.____
   A. variations in intensity of muscular contraction
   B. the number of fibers in the muscle which contract
   C. the circulation of blood within the muscle
   D. the manufacture of lactic acid in the muscle

42. In order to determine the basal metabolic rate of an individual, all of the following conditions must be included EXCEPT that the
    A. environment temperature must be comfortably warm
    B. test must be made from 12 to 18 hours after the last meal
    C. body must be in the waking state and at complete rest
    D. test should be preceded by a ten-minute period of vigorous exercise

43. Static and moving body postures are BEST judged on the basis of
    A. how well they meet the demands made upon them
    B. comparison with standardized charts
    C. muscular strength
    D. body flexibility

44. All of the following increase the efficiency of lifting heavy objects from the floor EXCEPT
    A. flexing the knees
    B. bending forward from the waist
    C. holding the object as close to the body as possible
    D. keeping the feet slightly separated both laterally and anteroposteriorly

45. All of the following associations are correct EXCEPT:
    A. Dorsal flexion – bending the foot at the ankle and elevating the front of the foot and toes
    B. Supination – turning the foot outward at its relation to the leg
    C. Plantar flexion – depressing the front of the foot and toes
    D. Adduction – turning the foot inward in its relation to the leg

46. All of the following concerning the Kraus-Weber Test for muscular fitness are correct EXCEPT:
    A. Failure on any one of the subtests classifies a child as a muscular-fitness failure.
    B. Flexibility in this test is measured by having the child bend forward slowly and touch his fingertips to the floor without bending his knees.
    C. The grip-strength test does not have much value since there is little relationship between grip strength and general body strength.
    D. The test measures large muscle groups of the upper and lower back, the abdominal wall and flexors of the hip joint.

47. Of the following, the one which is designed to reveal whether a child's growth is progressing properly in terms of his own body build is the
    A. Pryor Width-Weight Tables
    B. Wetzel Grid
    C. Quinby Weight Analysis Test
    D. Rogers Strength Index of Physical Fitness Index

48. The center of gravity of an individual of average build in an erect standing position is
    A. located in the pelvis in front of the upper part of the sacrum
    B. located at the articulation of the femur and the pelvis

C. located in the anterior wall of the pelvis
D. lower in men than in women because of anatomical structure

49. All of the following statements concerning lateral curvatures of the spine are correct EXCEPT:
    A. Some rotation of the vertebrae always accompanies lateral flexion of the spine.
    B. In a simple structural lateral curvature, the curve is confined to one region and there is no compensator curve.
    C. The shoulder on the side of a dorsal convexity is lower than the other shoulder.
    D. In a functional lateral curvature of the spine, the curve disappears when the individual suspends his body by hanging from the arms.

50. Vitamin A deficiency is associated with all of the following EXCEPT
    A. faulty development of the teeth
    B. impairment of vision in dim light
    C. impairment of epithelial tissue
    D. retardation in the development of bones

KEY (CORRECT ANSWERS)

1.	B	11.	C	21.	C	31.	D	41.	B
2.	C	12.	D	22.	C	32.	B	42.	D
3.	A	13.	D	23.	B	33.	C	43.	A
4.	A	14.	C	24.	B	34.	B	44.	B
5.	B	15.	B	25.	C	35.	B	45.	B
6.	B	16.	B	26.	B	36.	C	46.	C
7.	C	17.	D	27.	D	37.	A	47.	B
8.	B	18.	B	28.	A	38.	C	48.	A
9.	B	19.	B	29.	D	39.	D	49.	C
10.	A	20.	D	30.	A	40.	B	50.	D

TEST 2

DIRECTIONS: Each question or incomplete statement is followed by several suggested answers or completions. Select the one that BEST answers the question or completes the statement. *PRINT THE LETTER OF THE CORRECT ANSWER IN THE SPACE AT THE RIGHT.*

1. All of the following concerning a universal blood donor are correct EXCEPT that he
   A. is a person whose blood is of type O
   B. is one whose blood corpuscles are not agglutinated by the blood of anyone
   C. may give his blood to a person whose blood is type A or type B
   D. is the only type accepted for a blood bank

   1.____

2. Dried blood plasma can be made available for an emergency transfusion by the addition of
   A. a saline solution
   B. an alkaline fluid
   C. blood cells
   D. sterile distilled water

   2.____

3. All of the following are subjective symptoms EXCEPT a
   A. headache
   B. flushed face
   C. sore throat
   D. earache

   3.____

4. When taking the wrist pulse rate, one should avoid
   A. taking the pulse with the thumb
   B. counting the pulse beats for 1 minute, then checking the rate by counting for another minute
   C. having the patient support his arm and hand in a relaxed position
   D. taking the pulses on the thumb side of the wrist between the tendon and the wrist bone

   4.____

5. All of the following associations are correct EXCEPT:
   A. Etiology – science of the causes of diseases
   B. Sequela – abnormal consequence persisting after the recovery from a disease
   C. Prognosis – prediction of the duration, course, and termination of a disease
   D. Incubation – associated alterations of structure and functions during the course of a disease

   5.____

6. All of the following diseases are caused by a virus EXCEPT
   A. diphtheria   B. herpes   C. mumps   D. chickenpox

   6.____

7. All of the following destroy or inhibit microorganisms EXCEPT
   A. prophylactics   B. antiseptics   C. disinfectants   D. germicides

   7.____

8. All of the following associations are correct EXCEPT:
   A. Smallpox – rubeola
   B. German measles – rubella
   C. Mumps – infectious parotitis
   D. chickenpox - varicella

9. Of the following, the one NOT related to the other three is
   A. antidote
   B. antibody
   C. antitoxin
   D. antigen

10. In regard to rheumatic fever, it is CORRECT to state that
    A. it can be passed on from one person to another
    B. it is responsible for more heart trouble in children than any other cause
    C. once a child has had this disease, he is not liable to another attack
    D. there is a specific test for diagnosing the disease

11. Ringworm is caused by a microscopic
    A. mold
    B. worm
    C. yeast
    D. virus

12. All of the following associations of suffixes found in technical terms on a health record and meanings are correct EXCEPT:
    A. Osis – swelling
    B. Emia – blood
    C. Itis – inflammation
    D. Algia - pain

13. All of the following associations are correct EXCEPT:
    A. Active immunity – smallpox vaccination
    B. Passive immunity – diphtheria antitoxin
    C. Acquired immunity – resistance to another attack of measles
    D. Local immunity – resistance to a disease by a group of individuals within a limited area

14. All of the following statements are correct EXCEPT:
    A. The only carbohydrate found in the blood and used by the body is glucose.
    B. The liver is the great regulator of the blood sugar.
    C. The main storage house of excess carbohydrate stored in the body is the connective tissue.
    D. Glycogen is the term applied to the excess carbohydrate stored in the body.

15. All of the following are associated with the diffusion of digested foods EXCEPT
    A. arterioles
    B. capillaries
    C. lymph
    D. villi

16. All of the following statements are correct EXCEPT:
    A. More than half of the iron in the body is in the hemoglobin of the red blood cells.
    B. Iron deficient persons can absorb more iron from food than healthy persons.
    C. Iron is relatively high in foods of low moisture content.
    D. When the diet's supply of iron is in excess of body needs, it is stored in the liver for later use.

17. All of the following are associated with vitamin D EXCEPT
    A. ergosterol   B. sorbitol   C. calciferol   D. viosterol

18. The enzyme in the gastric juice that causes the curdling or coagulation of milk is
    A. renin   B. pepsin   C. rennin   D. lipase

19. Of the following, the one that is NOT associated with a lack of vitamins is
    A. beri-beri
    B. zerophthalmia
    C. trachoma
    D. night blindness

20. All of the following associations are correct EXCEPT:
    A. Folic acid – vitamin B
    B. Tetany – parathyroids
    C. Trypsin – gastric juice
    D. Insulin - pancreas

21. All of the following associations are correct EXCEPT:
    A. Vitamin E – antihemorrhagic
    B. Vitamin C – anti-scorbutic
    C. Vitamin B – anti-neuritic
    D. Nicotinic acid – pellagra preventive

22. All of the following forms of milk are comparable in food nutrients EXCEPT
    A. certified milk
    B. evaporated milk
    C. buttermilk
    D. homogenized milk

23. All of the following statements are correct EXCEPT:
    A. The presence of a sufficient quantity of fats in the diet does away with the necessity of using protein for fuel.
    B. Any considerable amount of fat in food eaten will slow down the digestion of the whole meal.
    C. The digestion of fats begins in the stomach.
    D. Layers of fat under the skin help to keep the body temperature constant.

24. All of the following are ductless glands EXCEPT the
    A. parotid   B. pineal   C. thymus   D. adrenals

25. Of the following, the tissue that has a capillary system is the
    A. dermis
    B. hair
    C. nails
    D. outer layer of skin

26. All of the following concerning a bursa are correct EXCEPT that
    A. it is a closed sac which contains a small amount of fluid
    B. its inner lining secretes fluid
    C. it prevents friction between muscles and underlying parts
    D. arthritis is caused by inflammation of the bursa

27. The body's CHIEF means of increasing heat production is by
    A. perspiring
    B. dilating the blood vessels
    C. shivering
    D. none of the above

28. With regard to nerve cells, the CORRECT statement is:
    A. They may be regenerated once they are destroyed in the body.
    B. They greatly increase in number after birth.
    C. They have a single axon and one or more dendrites.
    D. Messages may be transmitted either way between axons and dendrites.

29. The substance in the blood which plays a very important part in protecting the body against infection is
    A. heparin   B. cholesterol   C. properdin   D. hematin

30. The grouping of types of human blood is based upon the type of
    A. red corpuscles   B. thrombocytes
    C. platelets   D. white corpuscles

31. The contractions of the heart cause all of the following EXCEPT
    A. the arterial blood to move via the aorta to all parts of the body
    B. the lymph to move through the lymph capillaries into larger lymph vessels
    C. the venous blood to go to the lungs for oxygen via the pulmonary arteries
    D. intermittent changes in the shape of the arteries

32. All of the following concerning the epidermis are correct EXCEPT that it
    A. contains nerve fibers
    B. contains blood cells
    C. constantly renews itself by creating new cells which push upward
    D. can become thicker after a long period of constant rubbing and pressure

33. A patient who has acne should be advised to
    A. wash his face thoroughly at least twice a day with a mild soap and warm water
    B. apply a cleansing cream when retiring at night
    C. use a skin ointment with an oily base at night and in the morning
    D. squeeze the pimple or blackhead and apply iodine

34. All of the following concerning the feet are correct EXCEPT:
    A. The height of the arch is an indication of the strength of the foot.
    B. Arch supports are temporary expedients for the relief of foot pain.
    C. Neglected, weak feet become flexible flat feet.
    D. Rigid flat feet show depressed arches when the weight is not borne on the feet.

35. All of the following are deformities of the foot EXCEPT
    A. calcaneus   B. talipes valgus
    C. equinus   D. genu valgum

36. The INCORRECT association is:
    A. Endomorph – soft, round, tendency to lay on fat
    B. Somatomorph – tall, athletic, broad-shouldered
    C. Ectomorph – linear, fragile, delicate
    D. Mesomorph – square, rugged, hard

37. All of the following are important components of the visual act proper EXCEPT
    A. convergence   B. interpretation
    C. accommodation   D. fusion

38. The condition of the eye in which the eyeball is too long anterioposteriorly is known as
    A. ametropia   B. hypermetropia
    C. myopia   D. prebyopia

39. When the nurse tests students' vision by means of the Snellen chart, she is testing the students'
    A. peripheral vision   B. distance acuity
    C. near acuity   D. depth perception

40. All of the following statements concerning protein are correct EXCEPT:
    A. Protein is a source of energy.
    B. Protein is required for tissue building and repair.
    C. Vegetable proteins are generally as satisfactory as meat proteins in meeting body requirements.
    D. Cheese contains important animal proteins.

41. Foods rich in calcium and protein are also the BEST sources of
    A. iodine   B. phosphorus   C. copper   D. fluorine

42. A lack of thiamine in the diet may cause
    A. inability to see in a dim light
    B. lesions around the nose and eyes
    C. malnourishment of the bones
    D. impaired functioning of the digestive and nervous system

43. The food which is acid-forming is
    A. fruits   B. vegetables   C. meat   D. nuts

44. The LEAST desirable method of preparing vegetables is by
    A. adding baking soda to preserve the color
    B. steaming
    C. boiling for a short time in a small amount of water
    D. baking

45. A low-calorie diet should NOT be low in _____ content.
    A. fat   B. fluid
    C. carbohydrate   D. protein

46. Skim milk is rich in all of the following EXCEPT
    A. calcium   B. riboflavin   C. vitamin A   D. protein

47. Food allergies are due to sensitization to a
    A. carbohydrate   B. fat   C. mineral   D. protein

48. With regard to nutrition, the CORRECT statement is:
    A. Malnutrition is found only in low-income families.
    B. Obesity is generally due to faulty glands.
    C. Nutrition is affected by rest, recreation, and general mental health.
    D. Adolescents should take additional vitamin preparations in order to ensure adequate vitamin intake.

49. In order to improve the muscular state of the nation, it would be desirable to do all of the following for our youth EXCEPT to
    A. encourage participation in daily calisthenics
    B. promote participation in swimming
    C. popularize soccer as a game for school children
    D. emphasize competitive sports

50. The Menninger Foundation and Clinic is known for its work in
    A. posture
    B. nutrition
    C. mental health
    D. cancer research

KEY (CORRECT ANSWERS)

1. D	11. A	21. A	31. B	41. B
2. D	12. A	22. C	32. B	42. D
3. B	13. D	23. C	33. A	43. C
4. A	14. C	24. A	34. A	44. A
5. D	15. A	25. A	35. D	45. D
6. A	16. B	26. D	36. B	46. C
7. A	17. B	27. C	37. B	47. D
8. A	18. C	28. C	38. C	48. C
9. A	19. C	29. C	39. B	49. D
10. B	20. C	30. A	40. C	50. C

EXAMINATION SECTION
TEST 1

DIRECTIONS: Each question or incomplete statement is followed by several suggested answers or completions. Select the one that BEST answers the question or completes the statement. *PRINT THE LETTER OF THE CORRECT ANSWER IN THE SPACE AT THE RIGHT.*

1. A highly complex compound containing nitrogen essential for building and repairing of body cells and tissue is
   A. carbohydrates
   B. fats
   C. proteins
   D. vitamins
   E. minerals

   1.____

2. Which of the following is *generally* considered superior to other sources of basic amino acids?
   A. Fats
   B. Green leafy vegetables
   C. Poultry
   D. Fruits
   E. Milk, eggs and meat

   2.____

3. The building blocks for the manufacture of proteins in the body are
   A. amino acids
   B. carbohydrates
   C. fats
   D. thyroxin
   E. bile

   3.____

4. A *more highly* concentrated source of energy than either proteins or carbohydrates is
   A. hemoglobin
   B. vitamins
   C. sugars
   D. antibodies
   E. fats

   4.____

5. Two minerals related to the health of the bones are _____ and _____.
   A. calcium; phosphorus
   B. copper; zinc
   C. chloride; iodine
   D. fluorine; manganese
   E. sodium; iron

   5.____

6. A condition in which the blood is deficient in either quality or quantity of red blood cells is
   A. arteriosclerosis
   B. goiter
   C. schizophrenia
   D. anemia
   E. myxedema

   6.____

7. The CORRECT percentage of adult body weight in regard to water is most closely
   A. 35%   B. 45%   C. 50%   D. 60%   E. 75%

   7.____

8. The ability to do better physical labor may be achieved as a result of eating a breakfast containing both _____ and carbohydrates.
   A. vegetables
   B. minerals
   C. vitamins
   D. fats
   E. fruits

   8.____

9. The CHIEF reason for obesity is
   A. heredity
   B. overeating
   C. glandular
   D. psychological
   E. eating proteins only

9._____

10. The MOST effective method of determining sensitivity to food allergies is the _____ test.
    A. elimination
    B. patch
    C. skin
    D. Minnesota
    E. Salmonellosis

10._____

11. Of the following, the MOST sensible way to approach weight loss is to
    A. cut out breakfast
    B. cut out midday meals
    C. cut out dinner or evening meals
    D. discuss diet or weight-loss options with your physician
    E. drink less water

11._____

12. Control of bodily activities and movements is the responsibility of the
    A. nervous system
    B. endocrine system
    C. thyroid gland
    D. parathyroid gland
    E. skeletal system

12._____

13. The products of the endocrine glands are called
    A. hormones
    B. chromosomes
    C. eugenics
    D. pneumococcus
    E. toxins

13._____

14. Olfactory cells are important to us in regard to
    A. tasting
    B. touching
    C. hearing
    D. smelling
    E. production

14._____

15. The taste buds are embedded in the
    A. throat
    B. tongue
    C. teeth
    D. roof of the mouth
    E. esophagus

15._____

16. Excessive amounts of caffeine may result in
    A. indigestion
    B. nervousness
    C. sleeplessness
    D. irritability
    E. all of the above

16._____

17. On a camping trip, the BEST way to purify drinking water is to
    A. boil the water
    B. filter the water
    C. store the water in reservoirs and allow the impurities to settle
    D. chlorinate the water

17._____

18. Trichinosis is a disease that may result from eating insufficiently cooked
    A. veal
    B. pork
    C. mutton
    D. fowl

18._____

19. The normal temperature of the human body is _____ degrees.
    A. 68.0
    B. 90.6
    C. 98.6
    D. 99.4

19._____

20. The BEST treatment for a cold is to
    A. take a laxative
    B. go to bed
    C. exercise vigorously to work up a sweat
    D. gargle with salt water or mouthwash

    20.____

21. If sugar is found regularly in the urine, the disease that may be present is
    A. diabetes   B. anthrax   C. rheumatism   D. beriberi

    21.____

22. A psychiatrist specializes in the field of
    A. psychology
    B. infectious diseases
    C. high blood pressure and other circulatory diseases
    D. mental or emotional problems

    22.____

23. A person with persistent bad breath should
    A. clean his or her teeth several times daily to kill the odor
    B. have a medical examination to determine the cause
    C. gargle several times daily to kill the odor
    D. chew gum when with other people

    23.____

24. The BEST way for students to learn about health is by
    A. listening to their family and friends
    B. personal experience
    C. studying scientific facts
    D. seeking medical information on the internet

    24.____

25. Sensitivity to proteins contained in pollen, feathers, etc. may be the cause of
    A. tuberculosis   B. pyorrhea   C. arthritis   D. hay fever

    25.____

26. Identify the FALSE statement.
    A. Ability to drive a car is directly related to maturity and judgment.
    B. It is safe for a good swimmer to swim alone in a regular swimming pool.
    C. A pedestrian should walk on the left side of the road so that he will face the cars coming from the opposite direction.
    D. Carrying a passenger on a bicycle is not a safe practice.

    26.____

27. When a person who has been sick is recovering, he or she is said to be
    A. regenerating   B. anemic   C. convalescing   D. infectious

    27.____

28. The tuberculin test is helpful in determining which
    A. people are immune to tuberculosis
    B. people have been infected with tuberculosis germs and need additional tests
    C. people have recovered from tuberculosis
    D. part of the body is infected

    28.____

29. Of the following, the disease MOST likely to be fatal is
    A. mumps   B. chicken pox
    C. scurvy   D. tetanus (lockjaw)

30. Identify the TRUE statement regarding treatment of a fever by drinking whiskey.
    A. There is neither harm nor value in this method.
    B. The use of whiskey to treat a fever is standard medical practice.
    C. It is a little-known method but one that is frequently of value.
    D. It is more dangerous than helpful.

31. Food groups and the Food Pyramid are concepts related to
    A. the cultural significance of popular foods and beverages
    B. the nutritional value of eating different cuisines
    C. healthy eating and nutrition
    D. reducing calories

32. Identify the MOST accurate statement about the effect of alcohol on muscular coordination.
    A. An alcoholic drink just before playing a round of golf will increase a player's muscular coordination.
    B. The effect of alcohol on muscular coordination depends largely on the health of the individual.
    C. An alcoholic drink just before leaving a party will NOT decrease one's muscular coordination in driving an automobile.
    D. There is considerable evidence that the use of alcohol affects muscular coordination.

33. If an artery in the lower forearm has been cut, the pressure should be applied
    A. between the cut and the wrist
    B. either at the wrist or the elbow
    C. between the cut and the elbow
    D. both at the wrist and the elbow

34. Which of the following statements about posture is FALSE?
    A. Poor posture makes one appear less conspicuous.
    B. Carelessness is the cause of MOST poor posture.
    C. Poor posture increases fatigue.
    D. *Stand tall*, *Walk tall* and *Sit tall* are the chief rules for good posture.

35. Beriberi, rickets, scurvy and pellagra are examples of _____ diseases.
    A. circulatory
    B. nutritional
    C. communicable
    D. occupational

36. Which of the following statements about nutrition is FALSE?
    A. Most leafy vegetables are rich in vitamins and minerals.
    B. There is no harm in drinking orange juice and milk at the same meal.
    C. Eating fish is associated with improved brain function.
    D. Drinking more than six glasses of water daily is fattening.

37. Historically, another term used for poliomyelitis is
    A. tonsillitis
    B. goiter
    C. infantile paralysis
    D. spina bifida

38. The mineral needed by red corpuscles in the blood to help them carry oxygen is

   A. iron B. calcium C. fluorine D. phosphorus

   38.____

39. Emotional instability in adults is MOST frequently attributed to
   A. heredity
   B. heart conditions
   C. head injuries
   D. childhood home life

   39.____

40. Accidents due to _____ occur MOST often in the home.
   A. falls
   B. poisoning from drugs and cleansing materials
   C. burns and scalds
   D. gas poisoning

   40.____

KEY (CORRECT ANSWERS)

1.	C	11.	D	21.	A	31.	C
2.	E	12.	A	22.	D	32.	D
3.	A	13.	A	23.	B	33.	C
4.	E	14.	D	24.	C	34.	A
5.	A	15.	B	25.	D	35.	B
6.	D	16.	E	26.	B	36.	D
7.	D	17.	A	27.	C	37.	C
8.	D	18.	B	28.	B	38.	A
9.	B	19.	C	29.	D	39.	D
10.	C	20.	B	30.	D	40.	A

TEST 2

DIRECTIONS: Each question or incomplete statement is followed by several suggested answers or completions. Select the one that BEST answers the question or completes the statement. *PRINT THE LETTER OF THE CORRECT ANSWER IN THE SPACE AT THE RIGHT.*

1. Athlete's foot is caused by
   A. streptococcus   B. oxides   C. bacillus
   D. fungi   E. streptomycin

   1.____

2. An adult has _____ permanent teeth.
   A. 26   B. 28   C. 30   D. 32   E. 36

   2.____

3. Although some digested foods are absorbed by the bloodstream in the stomach, MOST absorption takes place in the
   A. liver   B. pancreas   C. gall bladder
   D. large intestine   E. small intestine

   3.____

4. The LARGEST gland in the body is said to be the
   A. liver   B. brain   C. heart
   D. stomach   E. large intestine

   4.____

5. Jaundice results from
   A. excessive amounts of bile being produced
   B. a shortage of lymph
   C. bile ducts being blocked
   D. an improper diet
   E. none of the above

   5.____

6. When the feces is slowed down in its passage through the colon, a condition of _____ is the result.
   A. diarrhea   B. hemorrhoids   C. indigestion
   D. constipation   E. jaundice

   6.____

7. Most stomach ulcers are caused by
   A. irregularities in heart beat
   B. varicose veins
   C. rapid peristaltic movement
   D. bacterial infection
   E. preference for spicy or acidic foods

   7.____

8. Sleeping pills typically contain
   A. marijuana   B. cocaine   C. antitoxin
   D. agglutinines   E. hypnotics

   8.____

9. The Schick test was a procedure used to determine if a person was immune to
   A. diphtheria   B. scarlet fever   C. typhoid fever
   D. tuberculosis   E. none of the above

   9.____

10. Most vaccines are made up of
    A. botulism
    B. trichinosis
    C. dead or weakened viruses or germs
    D. anthrax
    E. material from chicken eggs

    10.____

11. Tuberculosis is caused by a
    A. virus   B. toxin   C. bacteria
    D. genetic defect   E. toxoid

    11.____

12. Hydrophobia is a condition that has historically been associated with
    A. abnormal desire for water   B. rabies
    C. abnormal fear of darkness   D. drowning
    E. fear of heights

    12.____

13. Poor posture among school-age children is a(n)
    A. orthopedic defect   B. poliomyelitis defect
    C. osteomyelitis defect   D. epidemiologist defect
    E. none of the above

    13.____

14. _____ are generally not used for the diagnosis and/or treatment of cancer.
    A. X-rays   B. Radiation   C. Hormones
    D. Anticoagulants   E. Chemotherapy

    14.____

15. Hypochondria describes a person who
    A. fears the dark   B. daydreams
    C. imagines illnesses   D. fears water
    E. enjoys burning things

    15.____

16. Alcohol is one type of
    A. tranquilizer   B. pep pill   C. depressant
    D. stimulant   E. all of the above

    16.____

17. Ophthalmology is the medical field concerned with the
    A. ears   B. nose   C. throat   D. eyes   E. feet

    17.____

18. A basal metabolism test is taken to determine if
    A. the heartbeat is normal   B. the thyroid is functioning properly
    C. constipation exists   D. blood pressure is normal
    E. barbiturates exist in the blood

    18.____

19. The astigmatism test will determine a person's ability to
    A. see   B. hear   C. write   D. speak   E. reason

    19.____

20. A skin specialist may also be called a
    A. chiropodist   B. epidemiologist   C. dermatologist
    D. podiatrist   E. none of the above

    20.____

21. An electro-cardiograph
    A. photographs the kidneys
    B. charts heartbeats
    C. records blood pressure
    D. records reaction time
    E. photographs the lungs

22. Regular vigorous physical exercise will gradually
    A. increase the number of body muscles
    B. develop good character traits
    C. develop a heart condition
    D. increase heart efficiency
    E. weaken a person

23. Another name for hernia is
    A. laceration   B. groin   C. rupture   D. incision

24. All of the following are treatments for sudden onset of kidney stones EXCEPT
    A. surgery
    B. analgesics
    C. Flomax
    D. blood thinners

25. _____ is acted upon by bacteria in the mouth to produce acids that dissolve tooth enamel.
    A. Protein
    B. Ascorbic acid
    C. Sugar
    D. Phosphorus

26. Hemochromatosis is a condition in which excess _____ is stored in the _____.
    A. iron; liver
    B. calcium; kidneys
    C. lymph; pancreas
    D. bile; liver

27. An approved first-aid treatment would be to
    A. remove a foreign body from the ear with a match stick
    B. use a tourniquet to stop bleeding from a minor wound
    C. treat heat exhaustion with drinks that are high in salts or electrolytes
    D. apply absorbent cotton directly to a burn or scald

28. A blood count of a person suspected of having appendicitis reveals that the number of white corpuscles is normal.
    It may be concluded that the person
    A. probably has appendicitis
    B. probably does not have appendicitis
    C. is developing no resistance to fight a possible infection
    D. needs a blood transfusion

29. Artificial respiration is NOT applied for
    A. drowning
    B. gas poisoning
    C. corrosive poisoning
    D. electric shock

30. The term "enriched," as used on food labels, generally refers to bread made of white flour to which has been added
   A. milk, butter or eggs
   B. nutrients like thiamine, niacin and riboflavin
   C. protein, fiber and fat
   D. calcium, vitamin C and sugar

31. Fatigue due to sedentary or mental work is usually BEST relieved at the end of one's working hours by
   A. several cups of coffee
   B. eight hours of sleep
   C. a tepid shower
   D. recreational activity of a physical type

32. Which statement on alcohol and its uses is FALSE?
   A. Alcoholic beverages are useful in preventing and curing colds.
   B. Alcohol is to be avoided in the treatment of snake or spider bites.
   C. It is a mistake to take an alcoholic drink before going out in bitter cold weather.
   D. Alcohol has limited use as a medicine.

33. Normally, constipation is BEST avoided through the use or consumption of
   A. mineral oil   B. yeast
   C. laxatives   D. foods containing fiber

34. Though rare, tuberculosis cases should be considered primarily a result of
   A. poor nutrition   B. infection
   C. emotional ailment   D. hereditary disease

35. Gonorrhea is frequently a cause of
   A. stomach ulcers   B. insanity
   C. baldness   D. sterility

36. One purpose of a periodic health examination is the detection of all of the following conditions EXCEPT
   A. memory loss   B. heart disease
   C. cancer   D. high blood pressure

37. These hormones help to regulate various body functions. _____ is involved when we get excited or angry.
   A. Thyroxin   B. Adrenalin   C. Insulin   D. Pituitrin

38. To a person driving a car or riding a bicycle, peripheral vision is MOST useful for
   A. seeing better at night
   B. reading traffic signs more easily
   C. detecting moving objects at the sides
   D. judging more accurately the speed of approaching vehicles

39. Beer, wine and whiskey should be considered 39.____
    A. foods   B. tonics   C. stimulants   D. depressants

40. A good substitute for oranges as a source of vitamin C is/are 40.____
    A. tomatoes   B. beef
    C. cod liver oil   D. whole wheat bread

KEY (CORRECT ANSWERS)

1.	D	11.	C	21.	B	31.	D
2.	D	12.	B	22.	D	32.	A
3.	E	13.	A	23.	C	33.	D
4.	A	14.	D	24.	D	34.	B
5.	C	15.	C	25.	C	35.	D
6.	D	16.	C	26.	A	36.	A
7.	D	17.	D	27.	C	37.	B
8.	E	18.	B	28.	B	38.	C
9.	A	19.	A	29.	C	39.	D
10.	C	20.	C	30.	B	40.	A

TEST 3

DIRECTIONS: Each question or incomplete statement is followed by several suggested answers or completions. Select the one that BEST answers the question or completes the statement. *PRINT THE LETTER OF THE CORRECT ANSWER IN THE SPACE AT THE RIGHT.*

1. Digestion actually begins in the 1.____
   A. mouth
   B. pharynx or throat
   C. trachea
   D. stomach
   E. small intestine

2. Vomiting is USUALLY an indication that there is also a disturbance in some part of the body other than the 2.____
   A. stomach
   B. mouth
   C. throat
   D. small intestine
   E. large intestine

3. The normal breathing rate per minute for an adult is about 3.____
   A. 11 to 13
   B. 14 to 16
   C. 16 to 18
   D. 19 to 21
   E. 21 to 23

4. The MOST important to life is 4.____
   A. milk
   B. meat
   C. vegetables
   D. water
   E. fruits

5. Pneumonia causes an inflammation of the 5.____
   A. throat
   B. lungs
   C. stomach
   D. nose
   E. kidneys

6. The circulatory system does NOT involve the body's 6.____
   A. blood
   B. heart
   C. lymphatic vessels
   D. spinal cord
   E. blood vessels

7. To protect the body from infection and disease is the function of 7.____
   A. platelets
   B. white blood cells
   C. red blood cells
   D. hemoglobin
   E. gamma globulin

8. _____ carry blood away from the heart. 8.____
   A. Venules
   B. Veins
   C. Arteries
   D. Capillaries
   E. Descending vena cava

9. Defects that a person is born with are called 9.____
   A. endocarditis
   B. congenital
   C. cardiac
   D. rheumatic
   E. mutations

81

10. The MOST complicated system in the body is the _____ system.
    A. circulatory B. respiratory C. nervous
    D. digestive   E. motor

11. The autonomic nervous system controls
    A. voluntary muscles   B. smooth muscle
    C. conditioned reflexes   D. sympathetic movements
    E. involuntary muscles

12. *Spastic* is a term generally used in relation to
    A. nerves   B. muscles   C. emotions
    D. environment E. thoughts

13. The colored portion of the eye is called the
    A. cornea B. pupil C. iris D. sclera E. retina

14. Your _____ is NOT one of your body's weapons against germs.
    A. skin   B. hairs   C. nose
    D. antibodies E. phagocytes

15. Dizziness or faintness may be associated with a disturbance of the _____ system.
    A. nervous   B. respiratory
    C. circulatory D. all of the above

16. The LARGEST number of people are accidentally killed when
    A. swimming B. driving C. walking
    D. falling   E. flying

17. The LARGEST number of accidents occur
    A. at home   B. in the water   C. on the playground
    D. at airports E. on highways

18. Shock exists because of
    A. poor circulation of the blood B. rapid heart beat
    C. nervous tension   D. drop in body temperature
    E. open wound

19. A floor burn would be considered a(n) _____ wound.
    A. incised   B. abrasion C. laceration
    D. puncture E. bruise

20. A doctor uses a sphygmomanometer to test
    A. reaction time B. heart beat
    C. pulse rate   D. blood pressure
    E. amount of sugar in urine

21. Stuttering is USUALLY due to
    A. emotional disturbance
    B. nervous tension
    C. high blood pressure
    D. lack of muscular control
    E. childhood diseases

22. The capacity of the lungs and heart to carry on their tasks during strenuous activity is called
    A. muscle endurance
    B. muscle tone
    C. cardiorespiratory endurance
    D. respiration

23. A podiatrist is a specialist who treats the
    A. eyes   B. ears   C. feet   D. nose   E. mouth

24. Malignant tumor is associated with
    A. tuberculosis   B. heart disease   C. rabies
    D. moles   E. cancer

25. Skin pores can be found on all of the following EXCEPT
    A. arms   B. legs   C. palms   D. chest   E. feet

26. The chemical salt of _____, when found in drinking water or applied directly to the teeth, seems to help reduce tooth decay.
    A. chlorides   B. fluorides   C. sulphates   D. nitrates

27. When cold air or cold water hits the skin, the body reduces heat loss *principally* by
    A. expanding the pores in the skin
    B. generating more heat in the muscles
    C. reducing the size of the blood vessels in the skin
    D. making the heart beat faster

28. A cup of coffee with sugar but WITHOUT cream contains only
    A. vitamin B   B. calories   C. protein   D. fiber

29. A deficiency of _____ is a cause of night blindness.
    A. iodine   B. protein   C. vitamin A   D. vitamin C

30. MOST authorities believe the usual cause of color blindness is that it
    A. is an inherited characteristic, and so runs in families
    B. may develop from looking at brightly colored lights, especially red ones
    C. is a contagious infection caused by a filterable virus
    D. is caused by an injury to the eyes

31. Active acquired immunity occurs when a person has a disease and then recovers from it.
    This is common for the diseases of _____ and _____.
    A. tuberculosis; malaria
    B. measles; chicken pox
    C. colds; pneumonia
    D. diabetes; anemia

32. Fatty liver disease is commonly associated with
    A. alcohol consumption
    B. overproduction of bile
    C. a diet high in eggs and yogurt
    D. an imbalance in hormone production

33. If improperly maintained, forced-air heating systems in the home can cause a person to experience all of the following EXCEPT
    A. runny nose or congestion   B. dry mouth
    C. allergic reaction   D. pink eye

34. Antitoxin pertains to
    A. immunization
    B. sterilization
    C. germ-killing drugs
    D. determination of susceptibility to a disease

35. Someone experiencing hookworm was likely exposed through
    A. eating poorly cooked pork
    B. walking barefoot outdoors for prolonged periods
    C. an inadequate diet
    D. poor ventilation in the home

36. The most common reason a person is overweight is because they
    A. exercise improperly
    B. have inherited a tendency to be overweight
    C. have an underactive thyroid gland
    D. consume a high-calorie diet

37. A meal that consists of bread, macaroni, rice pudding and cake contains an excess of
    A. protein   B. vitamins
    C. carbohydrates   D. fats

38. Which statement about sunburn is FALSE?
    A. Sunburn is similar to any other burn and should be treated in the same manner.
    B. If a person who is badly sunburned develops a fever, a doctor should be called.
    C. A severe sunburn may be more serious than other burns of like extent.
    D. There is no danger of getting sunburned on a cloudy day.

39. Goiter may be caused by a lack of _____ in the diet or drinking water.
    A. iodine   B. chlorine   C. fluorine   D. bromine

40. It is FALSE that 40.____
    A. secondary sex characteristics generally become evident at adolescence
    B. the female reproductive organs which produce eggs are called ovaries
    C. the male reproductive organs which produce sperm are called testes
    D. girls and boys mature on the average at the same age

KEY (CORRECT ANSWERS)

1.	A	11.	E	21.	A	31.	B
2.	A	12.	B	22.	C	32.	A
3.	C	13.	C	23.	C	33.	D
4.	D	14.	C	24.	E	34.	A
5.	B	15.	D	25.	C	35.	B
6.	D	16.	B	26.	B	36.	D
7.	B	17.	A	27.	C	37.	C
8.	C	18.	A	28.	B	38.	D
9.	B	19.	B	29.	C	39.	A
10.	C	20.	D	30.	A	40.	D

TEST 4

DIRECTIONS: Each question or incomplete statement is followed by several suggested answers or completions. Select the one that BEST answers the question or completes the statement. *PRINT THE LETTER OF THE CORRECT ANSWER IN THE SPACE AT THE RIGHT.*

1. A state health officer is GENERALLY a
   A. specialist
   B. physician
   C. health educator
   D. member of the bar association
   E. nurse

   1.____

2. The SEVEREST forms of mental illnesses are classified as
   A. neurosis
   B. psychosis
   C. sublimations
   D. personality disorders
   E. peristalsis

   2.____

3. A public-health campaign educating people about blood pressure and circulatory health would likely include the definition of
   A. lymph nodes
   B. caloric intake
   C. hypertension
   D. red blood cells, white blood cells and platelets
   E. renal failure

   3.____

4. The appendix
   A. aids in elimination
   B. aids in respiration
   C. serves no function
   D. fights bacteria
   E. aids in digestion

   4.____

5. Diabetes is a disease of the
   A. pancreas
   B. kidney
   C. spleen
   D. gonads
   E. veins

   5.____

6. MOST all children are born
   A. with astigmatism
   B. nearsighted
   C. farsighted
   D. unable to hear
   E. blind

   6.____

7. Alcoholism is considered a
   A. habit
   B. disease
   C. sickness
   D. pleasure
   E. weakness

   7.____

8. Alcohol is absorbed directly from the
   A. small intestine
   B. large intestine
   C. stomach
   D. gall bladder
   E. kidneys

   8.____

2 (#4)

9. Anesthetics produce
   A. a feeling of warmth
   B. diseases
   C. a loss of pain
   D. freedom from diseases
   E. tuberculosis

   9.____

10. The PRIMARY fault of self-prescribed drugs is that they
    A. are too costly
    B. do not cure the cause
    C. are hard to get
    D. are too slow in acting
    E. weaken the taker

    10.____

11. Disease-producing bacteria form a poison called
    A. pimples
    B. toxins
    C. inflammation
    D. spores
    E. bacilli

    11.____

12. _____ diseases last for a long period of time.
    A. Chronic
    B. Cochlea
    C. Anaesthetic
    D. Analgesic
    E. Acute

    12.____

13. Rocky Mountain spotted fever is spread by
    A. ants
    B. dogs
    C. feces
    D. ticks
    E. flies

    13.____

14. Which word is NOT related to the others?
    A. Antitoxins
    B. Antibodies
    C. Phagocytes
    D. Vaccine
    E. Intravenous

    14.____

15. The MOST frequent cause of death is
    A. cancer
    B. nephritis
    C. tuberculosis
    D. heart disease
    E. skin disease

    15.____

16. A group of similar cells working together is called a(n)
    A. organ
    B. tissue
    C. nucleus
    D. nerve
    E. bine

    16.____

17. The contraction of striated muscle cells is controlled by the
    A. person
    B. nerves
    C. heart
    D. tissues
    E. cartilages

    17.____

18. The muscles are fastened to the bones at both ends by
    A. ligament
    B. ossification
    C. cartilages
    D. tendons
    E. coccyx

    18.____

19. The outer layer of the skin is called the
    A. callus
    B. dermis
    C. papillae
    D. epidermis
    E. cuticle

    19.____

20. Human eggs are produced in the
    A. vagina
    B. uterus
    C. ovaries
    D. fallopian tube
    E. conceptus

    20.____

3 (#4)

21. Heredity plays an important part in the transmission of   21.____
    A. cancer   B. color blindness   C. heart disease
    D. tuberculosis   E. streptococcus

22. Fatigue is produced by accumulations of dioxide and lactic acid in   22.____
    A. the muscle cells   B. lungs   C. respiratory system
    D. nerve cells   E. cardiac muscles

23. _____ is NOT a function of the bones of the body.   23.____
    A. Support   B. Attachment of muscles
    C. Manufacture of blood cells D. Protection
    E. Weight control

24. A hernia, or rupture, is more common in   24.____
    A. young girls   B. middle-aged women
    C. infants   D. men
    E. older women

25. The body's _____ glands sit atop the kidneys.   25.____
    A. adrenal   B. pituitary   C. thyroid
    D. parathyroid   E. pineal

26. An inflamed area containing pus is called a(n)   26.____
    A. blackhead   B. impetigo   C. pustule
    D. boil   E. fever blister

27. _____ is(are) the MOST important concerning vitamin D.   27.____
    A. Green vegetables   B. Lean meat   C. Sunshine
    D. Butter   E. Fruits

28. To recover from influenza, it is MOST important to   28.____
    A. rest and hydrate   B. move to a dry climate
    C. exercise by taking long walks   D. take antibiotics

29. Cooking vegetables by boiling decreases their nutritional value in respect to   29.____
    A. proteins   B. starch   C. vitamins   D. fats

30. The _____ destroy disease germs by surrounding and devouring them.   30.____
    A. red corpuscles   B. white corpuscles
    C. blood platelets   D. interstitial cells

31. An unconscious person should be given _____ as a first-aid measure.   31.____
    A. water   B. whiskey or brandy
    C. coffee or tea   D. none of these

32. The scientific name for the female reproductive cell is   32.____
    A. sperm   B. ovum   C. gamete   D. embryo

33. Little or no fiber is contained in
    A. raw fruits
    B. whole-grain cereals
    C. sugar and candy
    D. vegetables

34. The term *fracture*, as used in first aid, means a(n)
    A. bone out of joint
    B. broken bone
    C. injury to a cartilage
    D. severed tendon

35. A disease in which certain body cells seem to *grow wild*, thereby destroying the regular cells and tissues, is
    A. leprosy
    B. ulcers
    C. cancer
    D. hernia

36. It is NOT advisable to use cathartics and laxatives regularly because they
    A. weaken the muscle tone of the intestines
    B. destroy the enzymes of digestion
    C. cause one to lose appetite
    D. cause one to lose weight

37. Diseases that can be transmitted from one person to another by germs are
    A. infectious
    B. hereditary
    C. allergies
    D. non-communicable

38. From a health perspective, a campaign emphasizing the benefits of home fruit and vegetable gardens should focus primarily on which of the following?
    A. Harvesting techniques and timing for peak fruit ripeness
    B. The importance of properly storing and washing home-grown foods
    C. Amount of money saved on home-grown versus store-bought items
    D. Relationship between vitamin density and quality of soil mixes

39. The soft tissue that underlies the hard outer enamel of a tooth is called
    A. dentine
    B. cement
    C. connective tissue
    D. root

40. Which statement on the reliability and accuracy of health advertising over the internet and social media is TRUE?
    A. It is very reliable since it is vetted before being broadcast.
    B. It may be considered reliable since doctors often prescribe many of the health remedies advertised.
    C. Most of it is reliable and can be believed by the public.
    D. Much of it is of questionable reliability.

41. The *bends* is a(n)
    A. gymnastic movement
    B. disease of the intestinal tract
    C. disease of divers and caisson workers
    D. ailment due to inhaling dust

42. A condition that involves curvature of the spine is 42._____
    A. spinal stenosis   B. anemia
    C. rheumatoid arthritis   D. scoliosis

43. All of the following are procedures performed during the annual physical check-up of an overweight 30-year-old male EXCEPT 43._____
    A. blood test   B. urine analysis
    C. blood pressure reading   D. prostate exam

44. _____ applies to the destruction of bacteria. 44._____
    A. Quarantine   B. Vaccination   C. Disinfection   D. Inoculation

45. The age period in which lack of proper nutrition results in the MOST harm is 45._____
    A. from birth to 6 years of age
    B. childhood (approximately 6-12 years)
    C. adolescence (approximately 12-18 years)
    D. early maturity (18-24 years)

KEY (CORRECT ANSWERS)

1. C	11. B	21. B	31. D	41. C
2. B	12. A	22. A	32. B	42. D
3. C	13. D	23. E	33. C	43. D
4. C	14. E	24. D	34. B	44. C
5. A	15. D	25. A	35. C	45. A
6. C	16. B	26. C	36. A	
7. B	17. A	27. C	37. A	
8. C	18. D	28. A	38. B	
9. C	19. D	29. C	39. A	
10. B	20. C	30. B	40. D	

EXAMINATION SECTION
TEST 1

DIRECTIONS: Each question or incomplete statement is followed by several suggested answers or completions. Select the one that BEST answers the question or completes the statement. *PRINT THE LETTER OF THE CORRECT ANSWER IN THE SPACE AT THE RIGHT.*

Questions 1-9.

DIRECTIONS: Questions 1 through 9 are based on the following passage.

Astronomers have long argued whether a tenth planet, Planet X, exists in the solar system. Two astronomers presented their opinions. Astronomer 1 argued that Planet X does not exist, and Astronomer 2 argued that Planet X does exist.

Astronomer 1

The 4 terrestrial (smaller) planets - Mercury, Venus, Mars, and Earth - orbit near the Sun and consist mainly of heavier, denser elements. The 4 giant planets - Jupiter, Saturn, Uranus, and Neptune -orbit farther from the Sun and contain mostly lighter elements, which are gaseous on Earth. The ninth planet, Pluto, is smaller than the Earth, and its orbit is inclined from the common orbital plane of the other planets. Therefore, Pluto probably did not originate within the solar system, but was captured from outside. It is very unlikely that the solar system would capture 2 planets. It is also unlikely that Pluto could have been captured between the orbits of Neptune and Planet X if Planet X had been formed with the rest of the solar system.

Some astronomers cite the orbital deviation of comets to support the theory that Planet X exists. But the force of solar radiation or collisions with meteoroids could account for these deviations. Deviation in Neptune's orbit has also been used to try to demonstrate Planet X's existence. But undiscovered causes may account for this deviation. Finally, Planet X should also have caused deviation in Pluto's orbit. However, none has been discovered.

Astronomer 2

Even if Pluto had been captured, that would still not disprove the existence of Planet X. Pluto may once have been a moon of Planet X or Neptune. Planet X probably is 3 times more massive than Saturn and 1 1/2 times farther from the Sun than is Pluto. Only such a massive object could cause comets and the planet Neptune to deviate from their orbits. Finally, Pluto has completed only 1/4 of its orbit since its discovery. Astronomers may yet find a deviation in Pluto's orbit that would support the theory that Planet X exists.

1. According to Astronomer 2, if Planet X existed, it would PROBABLY be less massive than   1.____

   A. Venus
   B. Earth
   C. Mars
   D. none of the above planets

2. A comet would experience the GREATEST force of radiation when it was closest to

   A. the Sun
   B. the giant planets
   C. Pluto
   D. Planet X

3. Astronomer 1 implies that the 4 terrestrial and the 4 giant planets were formed

   A. at the center of the Sun
   B. in the immediate neighborhood of the Sun
   C. outside the solar system
   D. in the order of their distances from the Sun, from farthest to nearest

4. Concerning the orbital deviation of comets, Astronomers 1 and 2 DISAGREE about the

   A. existence of the deviations
   B. magnitude of the deviations
   C. nature of the force causing the deviations
   D. existence of the force of radiation

5. If a deviation were observed in the orbit of Pluto, the astronomer that would be MOST seriously challenged would be Astronomer _____ because such deviation would _____ .

   A. 1; have to be caused by meteor showers
   B. 1; have to be caused by a massive object
   C. 2; have to be caused by Neptune
   D. 2; prove Pluto is a captured planet

6. Jupiter and Mercury have similar

   A. orbital radii
   B. chemical compositions
   C. masses
   D. planes of orbit

7. On the basis of Astronomer 2's arguments, one could infer that a failure to view Planet X with a telescope could be due to the fact that Planet X is

   A. obscured by swarms of comets located far from the Sun
   B. hidden in Pluto's shadow
   C. located in a part of the sky that has not yet been carefully examined
   D. gaseous and absorbs light

8. Astronomer 2 implies that the deviation in the path of a comet would be caused by

   A. magnetic force
   B. gravitational force
   C. radiation from the Sun
   D. collision with another body

9. In the solar system, gravitational force is caused by the
   I. Sun
   II. giant planets
   III. terrestrial planets

   The CORRECT answer is:

   A. I only
   B. II only
   C. I and II
   D. All of the above

Questions 10-18.

DIRECTIONS: Questions 10 through 18 are based on the following passage.

To design an aircraft that can fly, engineers must solve certain basic problems. Today, engineers have computers and a large pool of knowledge to aid in the design of sophisticated aircraft. But the Wright brothers, Orville and Wilbur, used only a basic knowledge of physics and simple experiments to build the first powered aircraft, the Wright Flyer.

The Wrights hypothesized that an airplane must have a wing to generate *lift*, the upward force that offsets the weight of the airplane. The lift of a wing depends upon the area of the wing, the airspeed of the wing, the density of the air, and the *angle of attack* (the angle the wing makes with its direction of flight). But a moving wing also generates *drag*, the frictional force that resists movement. Drag increases as lift and airspeed increase. To overcome drag and to provide velocity to create lift, an airplane must generate *thrust*, the forward force provided in some aircraft by a propeller connected to an engine. To fly at a steady speed at a constant height, an airplane must maintain a balance among lift, weight, drag, and thrust. The Wrights used 2 wings in a biplane arrangement to provide lift and developed a light but powerful aluminum engine to create thrust.

Changing the direction of flight poses further problems. Simply moving the nose of an airplane to one side or the other will cause the airplane to make a broad skid turn. Its wings must *bank*, or tilt, in the direction of the turn before the airplane will change direction quickly. An airplane can be made to tip its nose up or down without climbing or diving by moving the *elevator*, a much smaller wing. This is done by changing the airspeed and thrust while increasing the angle of attack.

The Wrights made the Flyer bank by using cables that actually bent the wings. The Wrights believed that an aircraft must be unstable to change direction. They reasoned that the force necessary to turn a stable aircraft would be much greater than the force required to turn an unstable one. To make the Flyer unstable, the Wrights placed the elevators in front of the wings. The pilot had to correct any change in direction constantly or the change would rapidly increase. Later inventors learned that stable aircraft can easily change direction. As a result, modern airplanes are much simpler to control.

10. The forces acting on the airplane in flight are shown below.

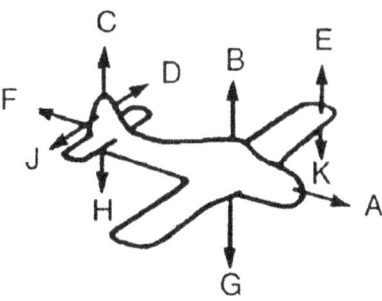

Which of these forces would have to be equal to each other in order to prevent the banking of the wings?

A. A and F
C. C and H
B. B and G
D. E and K

11. If the Wrights had wanted the Flyer to be stable, they PROBABLY would have

   A. placed the elevators behind the wings
   B. used 1 wing instead of 2
   C. added weight to the airplane
   D. increased the power of the engine

12. A conventional airplane that can fly at very low airspeeds MUST have a large

   A. wing area
   B. propeller
   C. amount of weight
   D. amount of drag

13. Both airplane and steamships use propellers. This fact indicates that both seawater and air

   A. have similar densities
   B. have similar chemical properties
   C. expand when heated
   D. flow readily under pressure

14. A certain modern aircraft with an engine approximately as powerful as that of the Wright Flyer can reach much greater speeds than the Flyer could.
   This difference in speed is due PRIMARILY to the fact that the modern aircraft has

   A. less drag
   B. greater drag
   C. greater lift
   D. greater weight

15. Which description of the forces acting upon a rocket rising vertically through the air must be TRUE?

   A. Drag is directed horizontally.
   B. Thrust is directed vertically.
   C. Thrust equals drag.
   D. Drag equals weight.

16. All winged aircraft have altitudes beyond which they cannot climb.
   This altitude limitation is due to the fact that as altitude increases, there is a decrease in

   A. drag
   B. gravity
   C. air density
   D. air temperature

17. An aircraft whose wings are much shorter than the length of the airplane was PROBABLY designed to

   A. carry large loads
   B. be unstable
   C. fly at high speeds
   D. fly at high altitudes

18. The fact that many aircraft can fly both upside down and rightside up demonstrates that lift depends upon

   A. drag
   B. the angle of attack
   C. banking the wings
   D. the weight of the airplane

Questions 19-33.

DIRECTIONS: Questions 19 through 33 are NOT based on a reading passage. You are to answer these questions on the basis of your knowledge in the natural sciences.

19.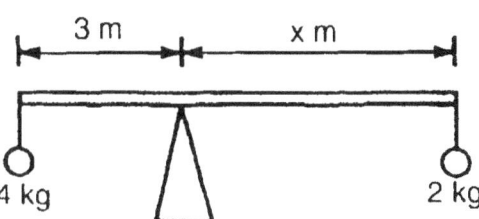

A uniform board of negligible mass is supported as shown above. A mass of 4 kilograms (kg) is suspended at one end, 3 meters from the point of support. A mass of 2 kilograms is suspended at the other end, x meters from the point of support.
If the board does NOT tilt, what is the length, in meters (m), of x?

A. 4 B. 6 C. 8 D. 12

20. A marble chip ($CaCO_3$) is dissolved in excess hydrochloric acid (HCl), and a gas is produced.
When the solution is evaporated, a white solid remains.
What is this solid?

A. Carbon (C)
B. Carbonic acid (H_2CO_3)
C. Calcium chloride ($CaCl_2$)
D. Calcium hydride (CaH_2)

21. A student places a cloth wick over the bulb of a thermometer, moistens the wick with water, and whirls the thermometer in the air.
The student is gathering data to calculate the
   I. air pressure
   II. wind speed
   III. relative humidity
The CORRECT answer is:

A. I only   B. III only
C. I and II   D. II and III

22. Which of these structures prevent MOST plant cells from bursting in a hypotonic solution?

A. Chloroplasts   B. Cell walls
C. Lysosomes   D. Ribosomes

23. The more complex plants (ferns, gymnosperms, flowering plants) can achieve a larger size and a more complicated organ structure than the less complex plants (algae, mosses, liverworts) because the more complex plants

A. have vascular systems   B. contain chloroplasts
C. are capable of mitosis   D. have cell walls

24. Two objects of the same volume are placed in 2 separate containers containing clear, colorless liquids. One object sinks to the bottom, but the other floats. Which conclusion concerning the densities of the objects and liquids could validly be made WITHOUT conducting further experiments?

   A. One of the objects has a greater density than the other.
   B. One of the liquids has a greater density than the other.
   C. The object that sinks has a greater density than the liquid it is in.
   D. The 2 objects and the 2 liquids are all of different densities.

25. Which of these facts does NOT support the theory of continental drift?

   A. The distance between North America and Europe increases yearly by a small amount.
   B. Igneous rocks of the seafloor increase in age from both sides of the mid-Atlantic ridge.
   C. Newly formed volcanic islands quickly become populated with living organisms.
   D. Coal has been found in Antarctica.

26. Which of these characteristics is NOT a typical mammalian feature?

   A. Body hair
   B. Three bones in the middle ear
   C. Internal fertilization
   D. Two-chambered heart

27. Suppose a membrane bag filled with iodine solution is placed in a beaker containing a starch solution. A blue-black color forms in the solution in the beaker, but NOT in the solution in the bag.
One can validly conclude that the membrane bag was

   A. impermeable to both starch and iodine
   B. impermeable to starch but permeable to iodine
   C. permeable to starch but impermeable to iodine
   D. permeable to both starch and iodine

28. A student measures the tension on a certain string and the frequency at which it vibrates. The resulting data are displayed in the table below:

Tension (newtons)	Frequency (cycles per second)
4	200
9	300
16	400

   Which equation accurately describes the relationship between string tension (T) and frequency (f)?
   f =

   A. $100\sqrt{T}$
   B. $\dfrac{100}{T}$
   C. $100T$
   D. $100T^2$

29. The noble gas neon is essentially chemically inert because its atoms

   A. form diatomic molecules
   B. bond together with triple covalent bonds
   C. bond together with highly charged ionic bonds
   D. have completely filled electron shells

30. Carbohydrates must be broken down into sugars before they can be absorbed by the human body.
   Which of these compounds does the body use to catalzye these reactions?

   A. Amino acids
   B. Fats
   C. Hormones
   D. Enzymes

31. Electrically neutral atoms of the Group IA elements, such as lithium, sodium, and potassium, all have equal numbers of

   A. protons
   B. neutrons
   C. filled electron shells
   D. valence electrons

32. An element with which of these electron configurations would be MOST reactive?

   A. $1s^1$
   B. $1s^2 2s\,2p$
   C. $1s^2 2s^2 2p^6$
   D. $1s^2 2s^2 2p^6 3s^2 3p^6$

33. If a 2.0 liter sample of liquid water at 100 Celsius is mixed with 1.0 liter of liquid water at 0.0 Celsius, what would be the APPROXIMATE temperature of the mixture, in degrees Celsius?

   A. 33
   B. 50
   C. 67
   D. 75

Questions 34-43.

DIRECTIONS: Questions 34 through 43 are based on the following passage.

All organisms exchange gases with their environments. Gases can enter or leave organisms only by passive diffusion across respiratory membranes. Whatever the life form, gases must be dissolved in the liquid covering the respiratory membrane before they can enter the organism.

Gas exchange surfaces in higher animals are generally formed by *evagination* - outward folding - or *invagination* - inward folding - of body surfaces. Aquatic animals usually have evaginated surfaces, such as gills. Oxygenated water constantly bathes these evaginated surfaces. As a bony fish swims, it forces water over its gills by opening and closing its mouth and gill flaps. Other aquatic forms have other methods of moving water over their gas exchange surfaces.

Land animals typically have invaginated gas exchange surfaces. The *tracheal system* of an insect is composed of a series of invaginated tubes leading from *spiracles* - openings on the insect's body - directly to the insect's cells. No cell is more than 1 or 2 cell layers away from the ending of a tracheal tube. Thus, oxygen diffuses directly into the cells instead of being transported by blood. The mammalian lung is another type of invaginated gas exchange surface. The lung is a highly branched series of invaginated tubes ending in sacs called *alveoli*. Each alveolus is surrounded by a network of capillaries. Oxygen in the alveoli dissolves in the moisture on the alveolar membranes and diffuses into blood cells in the capillaries.

There are exceptions to the general rule that aquatic organisms have evaginated gas exchange surfaces and land organisms have invaginated gas exchange surfaces. Sea cucumbers, for instance, have invaginated tubes that branch off the anal pouch. Water pumped into and out of the anal opening brings dissolved oxygen to the sea cucumber's respiratory membranes.

34. Individuals of certain fish species will die if prevented from moving through the water. The MOST likely reason why members of these species must keep moving is to

    A. keep their gills from invaginating
    B. supply energy for active transport of gases across respiratory membranes
    C. maintain pressure inside their tracheal tubes
    D. maintain a flow of water over their gills

35. Frogs can exchange gases through both their lungs and their

    A. hearts B. intestines
    C. trqcheal tubes D. skins

36. The hollow body of the hydra, a small aquatic organism, is a cylinder 2 cells thick. The hydra PROBABLY exchanges gases through

    A. gills
    B. sea cucumber-like tubes
    C. its entire body surface
    D. lungs

37. Crayfish have a pair of flat appendages located just in front of the gills. These appendages move back and forth continuously.
    To effectively exchange gases, crayfish, therefore, do NOT have to

    A. depend upon the passive diffusion of gases
    B. pump blood through their gills
    C. maintain a constant flow of water through their gills
    D. constantly move through the water

38. Which aquatic animal exchanges gases through an invaginated surface?

    A. Shark B. Whale C. Clam D. Lobster

39. A certain vertebrate changes from an aquatic adolescent into a terrestrial adult. During this metamorphosis, the animal's gas exchange system would MOST likely

    A. change from gills to lungs
    B. change from tracheal tubes to lungs
    C. remain unchanged as tracheal tubes
    D. remain unchanged as gills

40. Larval tiger salamanders growing in iodine-deficient water never reach the adult stage. Which of these gas exchange surfaces would be used by these larval salamanders for respiration?
    I. Gills
    II. Lungs
    III. Tracheal tubes
    The CORRECT answer is:

    A. I only
    B. II only
    C. III only
    D. I and III

41. A common feature of all gas exchange surfaces is

    A. a branched structure
    B. moisture
    C. the presence of capillaries
    D. the presence of tracheal tubes

42. A decrease in the rate at which a certain gas enters an organism could be caused by a(n)

    A. *increase* in the organism's metabolic rate
    B. *increase* in the amount of energy available for active transport
    C. *decrease* in the partial pressure of the gas in the environment
    D. *increase* in the partial pressure of the gas in the environment

43. Compared to concentrations of oxygen and carbon dioxide in the air, blood entering the lungs must have a(n) _____ concentration of _____.

    A. higher; oxygen
    B. equal; oxygen
    C. higher; carbon dioxide
    D. equal; carbon dioxide

Questions 44-50.

DIRECTIONS: Questions 44 through 50 are based on the following passage.

Color can be a useful tool in laboratory experiments. The absorption or emission of certain ranges of light wavelengths by ions or molecules causes color. The principal colors of light are red, orange, yellow, green, blue, and violet, each of which is associated with certain wavelengths. Other colors can be formed by the absorption or emission of combinations of these wavelengths.

Absorption of characteristic wavelengths of light by particles of *solutes* (dissolved substances) gives solutions their colors. Solution color is often affected by chemical reactions among solutes. *Oxidation-reduction reactions,* in which electrons are transferred among solute particles, can cause color changes. The addition of an acid or base to a solution also may produce a different color. An aqueous cobalt(II) chloride solution, for example, is red. In general, if an acid is added, the solution remains red. However, the addition of a base turns the solution blue and cloudy as cobalt(II) hydroxide forms and precipitates.

The colors of certain organic compounds known as *indicators* can be used to mark changes in the acidity of a solution. Some of the indicator molecules ionize in solution, and the resulting ions absorb different wavelengths of light than do the molecules. Since the ratio of ions to molecules depends upon the acidity of the solution, the color of the solution changes when the acidity reaches a certain known value.

In one method of *acid-base titration,* indicators are used to measure the concentration of a solution. A drop of indicator is added to a solution whose *molarity* (molar concentration, in moles per liter) is known. Small amounts of the solution of unknown concentration are measured into the known solution until the indicator changes color, marking neutralization. Using the molarity and volume of the known solution, the volume of the unknown solution used in the reaction, and the reaction equation, a chemist can determine the molarity of the unknown solution.

For example, suppose 500 milliliters of a sodium hydroxide solution of unknown concentration just causes the indicator in 1 liter of 0.01 M (moles per liter) sulfuric acid (H_2SO_4) to change color. Sodium hydroxide (NaOH) and sulfuric acid react according to the equation

$$H_2SO_4 + 2NaOH \rightarrow Na_2SO_4 + 2H_2O$$

The equation shows that twice as many moles of sodium hydroxide as sulfuric acid were used in the reaction. Since the sulfuric acid contained 0.01 mole of H_2O_4, all of which was neutralized, 0.02 mole of sodium hydroxide must have been used. The concentration of the sodium hydroxide solution is, therefore,

$$\frac{0.02 \text{ mole}}{500 \text{ milliliters}} \times \frac{1,000 \text{ milliliters}}{1 \text{ liter}} = 0.04M$$

44. Nitric acid (HNO_3 in aqueous solution) is colorless. An aqueous solution3of nickel(II) nitrate [$Ni(NO_3)_2$], is green.
These facts support the conclusion that the green color of nickel(II) nitrate is caused by _____ ions.

   A. nitrate
   C. nitrogen
   B. nickel(II)
   D. oxygen

45. Which of these procedures would distinguish blue light caused by emission from blue light caused by absorption?

   A. Projecting the light through a. colored solution
   B. Reflecting the light from a mirror
   C. Reflecting the light from the surface of water
   D. None of the above

46. If a drop of phenolphthalein is added to a beaker of aqueous sodium hydroxide, the solution becomes deep red. The addition of hydrogen chloride eventually causes the solution to become colorless.
This information supports the conclusion about phenolphthalein that it

   A. forms a precipitate when added to a base
   B. emits red light when added to a base
   C. is useful as an indicator in acid-base titration
   D. is decomposed by strong acids

47. Hydrochloric acid (HCl) and potassium hydroxide (KOH) react according to the equation shown below:

    HCl + KOH → KCl + H$_2$O

    Suppose 500 milliliters of 0.20 M KOH solution is exactly neutralized by 250 milliliters of HCl solution. What is the molarity of the HC1 solution?

    A. 0.10   B. 0.20   C. 0.40   D. 0.80

48. As water is added to a red cobalt(II) chloride solution, the solution color changes to pink. Which of these explanations of this color change is CORRECT?

    A. Less light is absorbed per unit volume of solution.
    B. Cobalt(II) and chloride ions bond with water molecules and absorb different wavelengths.
    C. Chloride ions absorb heat from water and emit pink light.
    D. Excess water causes cobalt(II) and chloride ions to bond, emitting pink light.

49. A certain indicator is colorless in acid and neutral solutions but turns blue in basic solutions. Suppose it is added to a solution, which remains colorless.
    The addition of which substance will change the color of the indicator?

    A. Ammonia   B. Carbon dioxide
    C. Hydrogen fluoride   D. Sulfur dioxide

50. The red color of a cobalt(II) chloride solution is caused by the cobalt(II) ion's

    A. emission of red wavelengths
    B. emission of all wavelengths except red
    C. absorption of red wavelengths
    D. absorption of all wavelengths except red

KEY (CORRECT ANSWERS)

1. D	11. A	21. B	31. D	41. B
2. A	12. A	22. B	32. A	42. C
3. B	13. D	23. A	33. C	43. C
4. C	14. A	24. C	34. D	44. B
5. B	15. B	25. C	35. D	45. D
6. D	16. C	26. D	36. C	46. C
7. C	17. C	27. B	37. D	47. C
8. B	18. B	28. A	38. B	48. A
9. D	19. B	29. D	39. A	49. A
10. D	20. C	30. D	40. A	50. D

SCIENCE READING COMPREHENSION
EXAMINATION SECTION
TEST 1

DIRECTIONS: Each question or incomplete statement is followed by several suggested answers or completions. Select the one that BEST answers the question or completes the statement. *PRINT THE LETTER OF THE CORRECT ANSWER IN THE SPACE AT THE RIGHT.*

PASSAGE

Photosynthesis is a complex process with many intermediate steps. Ideas differ greatly as to the details of these steps, but the general nature of the process and its outcome are well established. Water, usually from the soil, is conducted through the xylem of root, stem and leaf to the chlorophyl-containing cells of a leaf. In consequence of the abundance of water within the latter cells, their walls are saturated with water. Carbon dioxide, diffusing from the air through the stomata and into the intercellular spaces of the leaf, comes into contact with the water in the walls of the cells which adjoin the intercellular spaces. The carbon dioxide becomes dissolved in the water of these walls, and in solution diffuses through the walls and the plasma membranes into the cells. By the agency of chlorophyl in the chloroplasts of the cells, the energy of light is transformed into chemical energy. This chemical energy is used to decompose the carbon dioxide and water, and the products of their decomposition are recombined into a new compound. The compound first formed is successively built up into more and more complex substances until finally a sugar is produced.

Questions 1-8.

1. The union of carbon dioxide and water to form starch results in an excess of

   A. hydrogen   B. carbon   C. oxygen
   D. carbon monoxide   E. hydrogen peroxide

2. Synthesis of carbohydrates takes place

   A. in the stomata
   B. in the intercellular spaces of leaves
   C. in the walls of plant cells
   D. within the plasma membranes of plant cells
   E. within plant cells that contain chloroplasts

3. In the process of photosynthesis, chlorophyl acts as a

   A. carbohydrate   B. source of carbon dioxide
   C. catalyst   D. source of chemical energy
   E. plasma membrane

4. In which of the following places are there the GREATEST number of hours in which photosynthesis can take place during the month of December?

   A. Buenos Aires, Argentina   B. Caracas, Venezuela
   C. Fairbanks, Alaska   D. Quito, Ecuador
   E. Calcutta, India

5. During photosynthesis, molecules of carbon dioxide enter the stomata of leaves because

   A. the molecules are already in motion
   B. they are forced through the stomata by the son's rays
   C. chlorophyl attracts them
   D. a chemical change takes place in the stomata
   E. oxygen passes out through the stomata

6. Besides food manufacture, another USEFUL result of photosynthesis is that it

   A. aids in removing poisonous gases from the air
   B. helps to maintain the existing proportion of gases in the air
   C. changes complex compounds into simpler compounds
   D. changes certain waste products into hydrocarbons
   E. changes chlorophyl into useful substances

7. A process that is almost the exact reverse of photosynthesis is the

   A. rusting of iron   B. burning of wood
   C. digestion of starch   D. ripening of fruit
   E. storage of food in seeds

8. The leaf of the tomato plant will be unable to carry on photosynthesis if the

   A. upper surface of the leaf is coated with vaseline
   B. upper surface of the leaf is coated with lampblack
   C. lower surface of the leaf is coated with lard
   D. leaf is placed in an atmosphere of pure carbon dioxide
   E. entire leaf is coated with lime

TEST 2

DIRECTIONS: Each question or incomplete statement is followed by several suggested answers or completions. Select the one that BEST answers the question or completes the statement. *PRINT THE LETTER OF THE CORRECT ANSWER IN THE SPACE AT THE RIGHT.*

PASSAGE

The only carbohydrate which the human body can absorb and oxidize is the simple sugar glucose. Therefore, all carbohydrates which are consumed must be changed to glucose by the body before they can be used. There are specific enzymes in the mouth, the stomach, and the small intestine which break down complex carbohydrates. All the monosaccharides are changed to glucose by enzymes secreted by the intestinal glands, and the glucose is absorbed by the capillaries of the villi.

The following simple test is used to determine the presence of a reducing sugar. If Benedict's solution is added to a solution containing glucose or one of the other reducing sugars and the resulting mixture is heated, a brick-red precipitate will be formed. This test was carried out on several substances and the information in the following table was obtained. "P" indicates that the precipitate was formed and "N" indicates that no reaction was observed.

Material Tested	Observation
Crushed grapes in water	P
Cane sugar in water	N
Fructose	P
Molasses	N

Questions 1-2.

1. From the results of the test made upon crushed grapes in water, one may say that grapes contain

   A. glucose B. sucrose C. a reducing sugar
   D. no sucrose E. no glucose

2. Which one of the following foods probably undergoes the LEAST change during the process of carbohydrate digestion in the human body?

   A. Cane sugar B. Fructose C. Molasses
   D. Bread E. Potato

TEST 3

DIRECTIONS: Each question or incomplete statement is followed by several suggested answers or completions. Select the one that BEST answers the question or completes the statement. *PRINT THE LETTER OF THE CORRECT ANSWER IN THE SPACE AT THE RIGHT.*

PASSAGE

The British pressure suit was made in two pieces and joined around the middle in contrast to the other suits, which were one-piece suits with a removable helmet. Oxygen was supplied through a tube, and a container of soda lime absorbed carbon dioxide and water vapor. The pressure was adjusted to a maximum of 2 1/2 pounds per square inch (130 millimeters) higher than the surrounding air. Since pure oxygen was used, this produced a partial pressure of 130 millimeters, which is sufficient to sustain the flier at any altitude.

Using this pressure suit, the British established a world's altitude record of 49,944 feet in 1936 and succeeded in raising it to 53,937 feet the following year. The pressure suit is a compromise solution to the altitude problem. Full sea-level pressure can not be maintained, as the suit would be so rigid that the flier could not move arms or legs. Hence a pressure one third to one fifth that of sea level has been used. Because of these lower pressures, oxygen has been used to raise the partial pressure of alveolar oxygen to normal.

Questions 1-9.

1. The MAIN constituent of air not admitted to the pressure suit described was

   A. oxygen   B. nitrogen   C. water vapor
   D. carbon dioxide   E. hydrogen

2. The pressure within the suit exceeded that of the surrounding air by an amount equal to 130 millimeters of

   A. mercury   B. water   C. air
   D. oxygen   E. carbon dioxide

3. The normal atmospheric pressure at sea level is

   A. 130 mm   B. 250 mm   C. 760 mm
   D. 1000 mm   E. 1300 mm

4. The water vapor that was absorbed by the soda lime came from

   A. condensation
   B. the union of oxygen with carbon dioxide
   C. body metabolism
   D. the air within the pressure suit
   E. water particles in the upper air

5. The HIGHEST altitude that has been reached with the British pressure suit is about

   A. 130 miles   B. 2 1/2 miles   C. 6 miles
   D. 10 miles   E. 5 miles

6. If the pressure suit should develop a leak, the   6.____

   A. oxygen supply would be cut off
   B. suit would fill up with air instead of oxygen
   C. pressure within the suit would drop to zero
   D. pressure within the suit would drop to that of the surrounding air
   E. suit would become so rigid that the flier would be unable to move arms or legs

7. The reason why oxygen helmets are unsatisfactory for use in efforts to set higher altitude   7.____
   records is that

   A. it is impossible to maintain a tight enough fit at the neck
   B. oxygen helmets are too heavy
   C. they do not conserve the heat of the body as pressure suits do
   D. if a parachute jump becomes necessary, it can not be made while such a helmet is being worn
   E. oxygen helmets are too rigid

8. The pressure suit is termed a compromise solution because   8.____

   A. it is not adequate for stratosphere flying
   B. aviators can not stand sea-level pressure at high altitudes
   C. some suits are made in two pieces, others in one
   D. other factors than maintenance of pressure have to be accommodated
   E. full atmospheric pressure can not be maintained at high altitudes

9. The passage implies that   9.____

   A. the air pressure at 49,944 feet is approximately the same as it is at 53,937 feet
   B. pressure cabin planes are not practical at extremely high altitudes
   C. a flier's oxygen requirement is approximately the same at high altitudes as it is at sea level
   D. one-piece pressure suits with removable helmets are unsafe
   E. a normal alveolar oxygen supply is maintained if the air pressure is between one third and one fifth that of sea level

TEST 4

DIRECTIONS: Each question or incomplete statement is followed by several suggested answers or completions. Select the one that BEST answers the question or completes the statement. *PRINT THE LETTER OF THE CORRECT ANSWER IN THE SPACE AT THE RIGHT.*

PASSAGE

Chemical investigations show that during muscle contraction the store of organic phosphates in the muscle fibers is altered as energy is released. In doing so, the organic phosphates (chiefly adenoisine triphosphate and phospho-creatine) are transformed anaerobically to organic compounds plus phosphates. As soon as the organic phosphates begin to break down in muscle contraction, the glycogen in the muscle fibers also transforms into lactic acid plus free energy; this energy the muscle fiber uses to return the organic compounds plus phosphates into high-energy organic phosphates ready for another contraction. In the presence of oxygen, the lactic acid from the glycogen decomposition is changed also. About one-fifth of it is oxidized to form water and carbon dioxide and to yield another supply of energy. This time the energy is used to transform the remaining four-fifths of the lactic acid into glycogen again.

Questions 1-5.

1. The energy for muscle contraction comes directly from the

    A. breakdown of lactic acid into glycogen
    B. resynthesis of adenosine triphosphate
    C. breakdown of glycogen into lactic acid
    D. oxidation of lactic acid
    E. breakdown of the organic phosphates

2. Lactic acid does NOT accumulate in a muscle that

    A. is in a state of lacking oxygen
    B. has an ample supply of oxygen
    C. is in a state of fatigue
    D. is repeatedly being stimulated
    E. has an ample supply of glycogen

3. The energy for the resynthesis of adenosine triphosphate and phospho-creatine comes from the

    A. oxidation of lactic acid
    B. synthesis of organic phosphates
    C. change from glycogen to lactic acid
    D. resynthesis of glycogen
    E. change from lactic acid to glycogen

4. The energy for the resynthesis of glycogen comes from the

    A. breakdown of organic phosphates
    B. resynthesis of organic phosphates
    C. change occurring in one-fifth of the lactic acid

2 (#4)

    D. change occurring in four-fifths of the lactic acid
    E. change occurring in four-fifths of glycogen

5. The breakdown of the organic phosphates into organic compounds plus phosphates is an   5.____

    A. anobolic reaction   B. aerobic reaction
    C. endothermic reaction   D. exothermic reaction
    E. anaerobic reaction

TEST 5

DIRECTIONS: Each question or incomplete statement is followed by several suggested answers or completions. Select the one that BEST answers the question or completes the statement. *PRINT THE LETTER OF THE CORRECT ANSWER IN THE SPACE AT THE RIGHT.*

PASSAGE

And with respect to that theory of the origin of the forms of life peopling our globe, with which Darwin's name is bound up as closely as that of Newton with the theory of gravitation, nothing seems to be further from the mind of the present generation than any attempt to smother it with ridicule or to crush it by vehemence of denunciation. "The struggle for existence," and "natural selection," have become household words and everyday conceptions. The reality and the importance of the natural processes on which Darwin founds his deductions are no more doubted than those of growth and multiplication; and, whether the full potency attributed to them is admitted or not, no one is unmindful of or at all doubts their vast and far-reaching significance. Wherever the biological sciences are studied, the "Origin of Species" lights the path of the investigator; wherever they are taught it permeates the course of instruction. Nor has the influence of Darwinian ideas been less profound beyond the realms of biology. The oldest of all philosophies, that of evolution, was bound hand and foot and cast into utter darkness during the millennium of theological scholasticism. But Darwin poured new life-blood into the ancient frame; the bonds burst, and the revivified thought of ancient Greece has proved itself to be a more adequate expression of the universal order of things than any of the schemes which have been accepted by the credulity and welcomed by the superstition of seventy later generations of men.

Questions 1-7.

1. Darwin's theory of the origin of the species is based on

    A. theological deductions
    B. the theory of gravitation
    C. Greek mythology
    D. natural processes evident in the universe
    E. extensive reading in the biological sciences

2. The passage implies that

    A. thought in ancient Greece was dead
    B. the theory of evolution is now universally accepted
    C. the "Origin of Species" was seized by the Church
    D. Darwin was influenced by Newton
    E. the theories of "the struggle for existence" and "natural selection" are too evident to be scientific

3. The idea of evolution

    A. was suppressed for 1,000 years
    B. is falsely claimed by Darwin
    C. has swept aside all superstition
    D. was outworn even in ancient Greece
    E. has revolutionized the universe

1.___

2.___

3.___

4. The processes of growth and multiplication   4._____

    A. have been replaced by others discovered by Darwin
    B. were the basis for the theory of gravitation
    C. are "the struggle for existence" and "natural selection"
    D. are scientific theories not yet proved
    E. are accepted as fundamental processes of nature

5. Darwin's treatise on evolution   5._____

    A. traces life on the planets from the beginning of time to the present day
    B. was translated from the Greek
    C. contains an ancient philosophy in modern, scientific guise
    D. has had a profound effect on evolution
    E. has had little notice outside scientific circles

6. The theory of evolution   6._____

    A. was first advanced in the "Origin of Species"
    B. was suppressed by the ancient Greeks
    C. did not get beyond the monasteries during the millennium
    D. is philosophical, not scientific
    E. was elaborated and revived by Darwin

7. Darwin has contributed GREATLY toward   7._____

    A. a universal acceptance of the processes of nature
    B. reviving the Greek intellect
    C. ending the millennium of theological scholasticism
    D. a satisfactory explanation of scientific theory
    E. easing the struggle for existence

TEST 6

DIRECTIONS: Each question or incomplete statement is followed by several suggested answers or completions. Select the one that BEST answers the question or completes the statement. *PRINT THE LETTER OF THE CORRECT ANSWER IN THE SPACE AT THE RIGHT.*

PASSAGE

The higher forms of plants and animals, such as seed plants and vertebrates, are similar or alike in many respects but decidedly different in others. For example, both of these groups of organisms carry on digestion, respiration, reproduction, conduction, growth, and exhibit sensitivity to various stimuli. On the other hand, a number of basic differences are evident. Plants have no excretory systems comparable to those of animals. Plants have no heart or similar pumping organ. Plants are very limited in their movements. Plants have nothing similar to the animal nervous system. In addition, animals can not synthesize carbohydrates from inorganic substances. Animals do not have special regions of growth, comparable to terminal and lateral meristems in plants, which persist through-out the life span of the organism. And, finally, the animal cell "wall" is only a membrane, while plant cell walls are more rigid, usually thicker, and may be composed of such substances as cellulose, lignin, pectin, cutin, and suberin. These characteristics are important to an understanding of living organisms and their functions and should, consequently, be carefully considered in plant and animal studies

Questions 1-7.

1. Which of the following do animals lack?

    A. Ability to react to stimuli
    B. Ability to conduct substances from one place to another
    C. Reproduction by gametes
    D. A cell membrane
    E. A terminal growth region

2. Which of the following statements is false?

    A. Animal cell "walls" are composed of cellulose.
    B. Plants grow as long as they live.
    C. Plants produce sperms and eggs.
    D. All vertebrates have hearts.
    E. Wood is dead at maturity.

3. Respiration in plants takes place

    A. only during the day
    B. only in the presence of carbon dioxide
    C. both day and night
    D. only at night
    E. only in the presence of certain stimuli

4. An example of a vertebrate is the

    A. earthworm   B. starfish   C. amoeba
    D. cow   E. insect

5. Which of the following statements is true?   5.____

   A. All animals eat plants as a source of food.
   B. Respiration, in many ways, is the reverse of photo-synthesis.
   C. Man is an invertebrate animal.
   D. Since plants have no hearts, they can not develop high pressures in their cells.
   E. Plants can not move.

6. Which of the following do plants lack?   6.____

   A. A means of movement
   B. Pumping structures
   C. Special regions of growth
   D. Reproduction by gametes
   E. A digestive process

7. A substance that can be synthesized by green plants but NOT by animals is   7.____

   A. protein   B. cellulose   C. carbon dioxide
   D. uric acid   E. water

TEST 7

DIRECTIONS: Each question or incomplete statement is followed by several suggested answers or completions. Select the one that BEST answers the question or completes the statement. *PRINT THE LETTER OF THE CORRECT ANSWER IN THE SPACE AT THE RIGHT.*

PASSAGE

Sodium chloride, being by far the largest constituent of the mineral matter of the blood, assumes special significance in the regulation of water exchanges in the organism. And, as Cannon has emphasized repeatedly, these latter are more extensive and more important than may at first thought appear. He points out "there are a number of circulations of the fluid out of the body and back again, without loss." Thus, by example, it is estimated that from a quart and one-half of water daily "leaves the body" when it enters the mouth as saliva; another one or two quarts are passed out as gastric juice; and perhaps the same amount is contained in the bile and the secretions of the pancreas and the intestinal wall. This large volume of water enters the digestive processes; and practically all of it is reabsorbed through the intestinal wall, where it performs the equally important function of carrying in the digested foodstuffs. These and other instances of what Cannon calls "the conservative use of water in our bodies" involve essentially osmotic pressure relationships in which the concentration of sodium chloride plays an important part.

Questions 1-11.

1. This passage implies that

    A. the contents of the alimentary canal are not to be considered within the body
    B. sodium chloride does not actually enter the body
    C. every particle of water ingested is used over and over again
    D. water can not be absorbed by the body unless it contains sodium chloride
    E. substances can pass through the intestinal wall in only one direction

2. According to this passage, which of the following processes requires MOST water? The

    A. absorption of digested foods
    B. secretion of gastric juice
    C. secretion of saliva
    D. production of bile
    E. concentration of sodium chloride solution

3. A body fluid that is NOT saline is

    A. blood   B. urine   C. bile
    D. gastric juice   E. saliva

4. An organ that functions as a storage reservoir from which large quantities of water are reabsorbed into the body is the

    A. kidney   B. liver   C. large intestine
    D. mouth   E. pancreas

5. Water is reabsorbed into the body by the process of

   A. secretion B. excretion C. digestion
   D. osmosis E. oxidation

6. Digested food enters the body PRINCIPALLY through the

   A. mouth B. liver C. villi
   D. pancreas E. stomach

7. The metallic element found in the blood in compound form and present there in larger quantities than any other metallic element is

   A. iron B. calcium C. magnesium
   D. chlorine E. sodium

8. An organ that removes water from the body and prevents its reabsorption for use in the body processes is the

   A. pancreas B. liver C. small intestine
   D. lungs E. large intestine

9. In which of the following processes is sodium chloride removed MOST rapidly from the body?

   A. Digestion B. Breathing C. Oxidation
   D. Respiration E. Perspiration

10. Which of the following liquids would pass from the alimentary canal into the blood MOST rapidly?

    A. A dilute solution of sodium chloride in water
    B. Gastric juice
    C. A concentrated solution of sodium chloride in water
    D. Digested food
    E. Distilled water

11. The reason why it is unsafe to drink ocean water even under conditions of extreme thirst is that it

    A. would reduce the salinity of the blood to a dangerous level
    B. contains dangerous disease germs
    C. contains poisonous salts
    D. would greatly increase the salinity of the blood
    E. would cause salt crystals to form in the blood stream

TEST 8

DIRECTIONS: Each question or incomplete statement is followed by several suggested answers or completions. Select the one that BEST answers the question or completes the statement. *PRINT THE LETTER OF THE CORRECT ANSWER IN THE SPACE AT THE RIGHT.*

PASSAGE

The discovery of antitoxin and its specific antagonistic effect upon toxin furnished an opportunity for the accurate investigation of the relationship of a bacterial antigen and its antibody. Toxin-antitoxin reactions were the first immunological processes to which experimental precision could be applied, and the discovery of principles of great importance resulted from such studies. A great deal of the work was done with diphtheria toxin and antitoxin and the facts elucidated with these materials are in principle applicable to similar substances.

The simplest assumption to account for the manner in which an antitoxin renders a toxin innocuous would be that the antitoxin destroys the toxin. Roux and Buchner, however, advanced the opinion that the antitoxin did not act directly upon the toxin, but affected it indirectly through the mediation of tissue cells. Ehrlich, on the other hand, conceived the reaction of toxin and antitoxin as a direct union, analogous to the chemical neutralization of an acid by a base.

The conception of toxin destruction was conclusively refuted by the experiments of Calmette. This observer, working with snake poison, found that the poison itself (unlike most other toxins) possessed the property of resisting heat to 100 degrees C, while its specific antitoxin, like other antitoxins, was destroyed at or about 70 degrees C. Nontoxic mixtures of the two substanues, when subjected to heat, regained their toxic properties. The natural inference from these observations was that the toxin in the original mixture had not been destroyed, but had been merely inactiviated by the presence of the antitoxin and again set free after destruction of the antitoxin by heat.

Questions 1-10.

1. Both toxins and antitoxins ORDINARILY

    A. are completely destroyed at body temperatures
    B. are extremely resistant to heat
    C. can exist only in combination
    D. are destroyed at 180° F
    E. are products of nonliving processes

2. MOST toxins can be destroyed by

    A. bacterial action
    B. salt solutions
    C. boiling
    D. diphtheria antitoxin
    E. other toxins

3. Very few disease organisms release a true toxin into the blood stream. It would follow, then, that

    A. studies of snake venom reactions have no value
    B. studies of toxin-antitoxin reactions are of little importance

C. the treatment of most diseases must depend upon information obtained from study of a few
D. antitoxin plays an important part in the body defense against the great majority of germs
E. only toxin producers are dangerous

4. A person becomes susceptible to infection again immediately after recovering from   4.____

   A. mumps   B. tetanus   C. diphtheria
   D. smallpox   E. tuberculosis

5. City people are more frequently immune to communicable diseases than country people are because   5.____

   A. country people eat better food
   B. city doctors are better than country doctors
   C. the air is more healthful in the country
   D. country people have fewer contacts with disease carriers
   E. there are more doctors in the city than in the country

6. The substances that provide us with immunity to disease are found in the body in the   6.____

   A. blood serum   B. gastric juice   C. urine
   D. white blood cells   E. red blood cells

7. A person ill with diphtheria would MOST likely be treated with   7.____

   A. diphtheria toxin   B. diphtheria toxoid
   C. dead diphtheria germs   D. diphtheria antitoxin
   E. live diphtheria germs

8. To determine susceptibility to diphtheria, an individual may be given the   8.____

   A. Wassermann test   B. Schick test
   C. Widal test   D. Dick test
   E. Kahn test

9. Since few babies under six months of age contract diphtheria, young babies PROBABLY   9.____

   A. are never exposed to diphtheria germs
   B. have high body temperatures that destroy the toxin if acquired
   C. acquire immunity from their mothers
   D. acquire immunity from their fathers
   E. are too young to become infected

10. Calmette's findings   10.____

    A. contradicted both Roux and Buchner's opinion and Ehrlich's conception
    B. contradicted Roux and Buchner, but supported Ehrlich
    C. contradicted Ehrlich, but supported Roux and Buchner
    D. were consistent with both theories
    E. had no bearing on the point at issue

TEST 9

DIRECTIONS: Each question or incomplete statement is followed by several suggested answers or completions. Select the one that BEST answers the question or completes the statement. *PRINT THE LETTER OF THE CORRECT ANSWER IN THE SPACE AT THE RIGHT.*

PASSAGE

In the days of sailing ships, when voyages were long and uncertain, provisions for many months were stored without refrigeration in the holds of the ships. Naturally no fresh or perishable foods could be included. Toward the end of particularly long voyages the crews of such ships became ill and often many died from scurvy. Many men, both scientific and otherwise, tried to devise a cure for scurvy. Among the latter was John Hall, a son-in-law of William Shakespeare, who cured some cases of scurvy by administering a sour brew made from scurvy grass and water cress.

The next step was the suggestion of William Harvey that scurvy could be prevented by giving the men lemon juice. He thought that the beneficial substance was the acid contained in the fruit.

The third step was taken by Dr. James Lind, an English naval surgeon, who performed the following experiment with 12 sailors, all of whom were sick with scurvy: Each was given the same diet, except that four of the men received small amounts of dilute sulfuric acid, four others were given vinegar and the remaining four were given lemons. Only those who received the fruit recovered.

Questions 1-7.

1. Credit for solving the problem described above belongs to

    A. Hall, because he first devised a cure for scurvy
    B. Harvey, because he first proposed a solution of the problem
    C. Lind, because he proved the solution by means of an experiment
    D. both Harvey and Lind, because they found that lemons are more effective than scurvy grass or water cress
    E. all three men, because each made some contribution

2. A good substitute for lemons in the treatment of scurvy is

    A. fresh eggs   B. tomato juice   C. cod-liver oil
    D. liver   E. whole-wheat bread

3. The number of control groups that Dr. Lind used in his experiment was

    A. one   B. two   C. three   D. four   E. none

4. A substance that will turn blue litmus red is

    A. aniline   B. lye   C. ice
    D. vinegar   E. table salt

5. The hypothesis tested by Lind was:

    A. Lemons contain some substance not present in vinegar.
    B. Citric acid is the most effective treatment for scurvy.

- C. Lemons contain some unknown acid that will cure scurvy.
- D. Some specific substance, rather than acids in general, is needed to cure scurvy.
- E. The substance needed to cure scurvy is found only in lemons.

6. A problem that Lind's experiment did NOT solve was: 6.____

   - A. Will citric acid alone cure scurvy?
   - B. Will lemons cure scurvy?
   - C. Will either sulfuric acid or vinegar cure scurvy?
   - D. Are all substances that contain acids equally effective as a treatment for scurvy?
   - E. Are lemons more effective than either vinegar or sulfuric acid in the treatment of scurvy?

7. The PRIMARY purpose of a controlled scientific experiment is to   7.____

   - A. get rid of superstitions
   - B. prove a hypothesis is correct
   - C. disprove a theory that is false
   - D. determine whether a hypothesis is true or false
   - E. discover new facts

TEST 10

DIRECTIONS: Each question or incomplete statement is followed by several suggested answers or completions. Select the one that BEST answers the question or completes the statement. *PRINT THE LETTER OF THE CORRECT ANSWER IN THE SPACE AT THE RIGHT.*

PASSAGE

The formed elements of the blood are the red corpuscles or erythrocytes, the white corpuscles or leucocytes, the blood platelets, and the so-called blood dust or hemoconiae. Together, these constitute 30-40 per cent by volume of the whole blood, the remainder being taken up by the plasma. In man, there are normally 5,000,000 red cells per cubic millimeter of blood; the count is somewhat lower in women. Variations occur frequently, especially after exercise or a heavy meal, or at high altitudes. Except in camels, which have elliptical corpuscles, the shape of the mammalian corpuscle is that of a circular, nonnucleated, bi-concave disk. The average diameter usually given is 7.7 microns, a value obtained by examining dried preparations of blood and considered by Ponder to be too low. Ponder's own observations, made on red cells in the fresh state, show the human corpuscle to have an average diameter of 8.8 microns. When circulating in the blood vessels, the red cell does not maintain a fixed shape but changes its form constantly, especially in the small capillaries. The red blood corpuscles are continually undergoing destruction, new corpuscles being formed to replace them. The average life of red corpuscles has been estimated by various investigators to be between three and six weeks. Preceding destruction, changes in the composition of the cells are believed to occur which render them less resistant. In the process of destruction, the lipids of the membrane are dissolved and the hemoglobin which is liberated is the most important, though probably not the only, source of bilirubin. The belief that the liver is the only site of red cell destruction is no longer generally held. The leucocytes, of which there are several forms, usually number between 7000 and 9000 per cubic millimeter of blood. These increase in number in disease, particularly when there is bacterial infection.

Questions 1-10.

1. Leukemia is a disease involving the

    A. red cells
    B. white cells
    C. plasma
    D. blood platelets
    E. blood dust

2. Are the erythrocytes in the blood increased in number after a heavy meal? The paragraph implies that this

    A. is true
    B. holds only for camels
    C. is not true
    D. may be true
    E. depends on the number of white cells

3. When blood is dried, the red cells

    A. contract
    B. remain the same size
    C. disintegrate
    D. expand
    E. become elliptical

4. Ponder is probably classified as a professional

    A. pharmacist
    B. physicist
    C. psychologist
    D. physiologist
    E. psychiatrist

5. The term "erythema" when applied to skin conditions signifies

   A. redness
   B. swelling
   C. irritation
   D. pain
   E. roughness

6. Lipids are insoluble in water and soluble in such solvents as ether, chloroform and benzene. It may be inferred that the membranes of red cells MOST closely resemble

   A. egg white
   B. sugar
   C. bone
   D. butter
   E. cotton fiber

7. Analysis of a sample of blood yields cell counts of 4,800,000 erythrocytes and 16,000 leucocytes per cubic millimeter. These data suggest that the patient from whom the blood was taken

   A. is anemic
   B. has been injuriously invaded by germs
   C. has been exposed to high-pressure air
   D. has a normal cell count
   E. has lost a great deal of blood

8. Bilirubin, a bile pigment, is

   A. an end product of several different reactions
   B. formed only in the liver
   C. formed from the remnants of the cell membranes of erythrocytes
   D. derived from hemoglobin exclusively
   E. a precursor of hemoglobin

9. Bancroft found that the blood count of the natives in the Peruvian Andes differed from that usually accepted as normal. The blood PROBABLY differed in respect to

   A. leucocytes
   B. blood platelets
   C. cell shapes
   D. erythrocytes
   E. hemoconiae

10. Hemoglobin is probably NEVER found

    A. free in the blood stream
    B. in the red cells
    C. in women's blood
    D. in the blood after exercise
    E. in the leucocytes

TEST 11

Questions 1-7.

DIRECTIONS: Each question or incomplete statement is followed by several suggested answers or completions. Select the one that BEST answers the question or completes the statement. *PRINT THE LETTER OF THE CORRECT ANSWER IN THE SPACE AT THE RIGHT.*

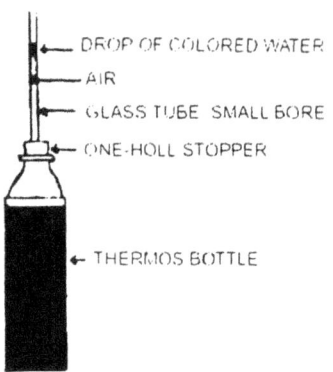

1. The device shown in the diagram above indicates changes that are measured more accurately by a(n)

    A. thermometer   B. hygrometer   C. anemometer
    D. hydrometer   E. barometer

    1.___

2. If the device is placed in a cold refrigerator for 72 hours, which of the following is MOST likely to happen?

    A. The stopper will be forced out of the bottle.
    B. The drop of water will evaporate.
    C. The drop will move downward.
    D. The drop will move upward.
    E. No change will take place.

    2.___

3. When the device was carried in an elevator from the first floor to the sixth floor of a building, the drop of colored water moved about 1/4 inch in the tube. Which of the following is MOST probably true? The drop moved

    A. *downward* because there was a decrease in the air pressure
    B. *upward* because there was a decrease in the air pressure
    C. *downward* because there was an increase in the air temperature
    D. *upward* because there was an increase in the air temperature
    E. *downward* because there was an increase in the temperature and a decrease in the pressure

    3.___

4. The part of a thermos bottle into which liquids are poured consists of

    A. a single-walled, metal flask coated with silver
    B. two flasks, one of glass and one of silvered metal
    C. two silvered-glass flasks separated by a vacuum
    D. two silver flasks separated by a vacuum
    E. a single-walled, glass flask with a silver-colored coating

    4.___

5. The thermos bottle is MOST similar in principle to

   A. the freezing unit in an electric refrigerator
   B. radiant heaters
   C. solar heating systems
   D. storm windows
   E. a thermostatically controlled heating system

6. In a plane flying at an altitude where the air pressure is only half the normal pressure at sea level, the plane's altimeter should read, *approximately,*

   A. 3000 feet B. 9000 feet C. 18000 feet
   D. 27000 feet E. 60000 feet

7. Which of the following is the POOREST conductor of heat?

   A. Air under a pressure of 1.5 pounds per square inch
   B. Air under a pressure of 15 pounds per square inch
   C. Unsilvered glass
   D. Silvered glass
   E. Silver

TEST 12

DIRECTIONS: Each question or incomplete statement is followed by several suggested answers or completions. Select the one that BEST answers the question or completes the statement. *PRINT THE LETTER OF THE CORRECT ANSWER IN THE SPACE AT THE RIGHT.*

PASSAGE

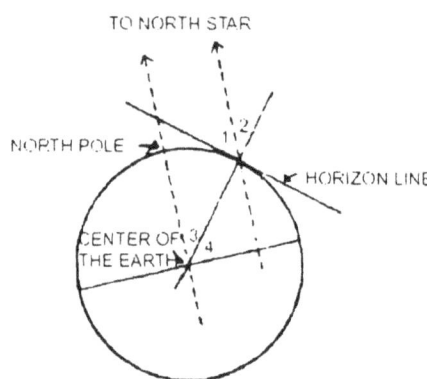

The latitude of any point on the earth's surface is the angle between a plumb line dropped to the center of the earth from that point and the plane of the earth's equator. Since it is impossible to go to the center of the earth to measure latitude, the latitude of any point may be determined indirectly as shown in the accompanying diagram.

It will be recalled that the axis of the earth, if extended outward, passes very near the North Star. Since the North Star is, for all practical purposes, infinitely distant, the line of sight to the North Star of an observer on the surface of the earth is virtually parallel with the earth's axis. Angle 1, then, in the diagram represents the angular distance of the North Star above the horizon. Angle 2 is equal to angle 3, because when two parallel lines are intersected by a straight line, the corresponding angles are equal. Angle 1 plus angle 2 is a right angle and so is angle 3 plus angle 4. Therefore, angle 1 equals angle 4 because when equals are subtracted from equals the results are equal.

Questions 1-10.

1. If an observer finds that the angular distance of the North Star above the horizon is 30, his latitude is   1.___

    A. 15° N   B. 30° N   C. 60° N   D. 90° N   E. 120° N

2. To an observer on the equator, the North Star would be   2.___

    A. 30° above the horizon   B. 60° above the horizon
    C. 90° above the horizon   D. on the horizon
    E. below the horizon

124

3. To an observer on the Arctic Circle, the North Star would be

   A. directly overhead
   B. 23 1/2° above the horizon
   C. 66 1/2° above the horizon
   D. on the horizon
   E. below the horizon

4. The distance around the earth along a certain parallel of latitude is 3600 miles. At that latitude, how many miles are there in one degree of longitude?

   A. 1 mile   B. 10 miles   C. 30 miles
   D. 69 miles   E. 100 miles

5. At which of the following latitudes would the sun be DIRECTLY overhead at noon on June 21?

   A. 0°   B. 23 1/2°S   C. 23 1/2°N
   D. 66 1/2°N   E. 66 1/2°S

6. On March 21 the number of hours of daylight at places on the Arctic Circle is

   A. none   B. 8   C. 12   D. 16   E. 24

7. The distance from the equator to the 45th parallel, measured along a meridian, is, *approximately,*

   A. 450 miles   B. 900 miles   C. 1250 miles
   D. 3125 miles   E. 6250 miles

8. The difference in time between the meridians that pass through longitude 45°E and longitude 105°W

   A. 6 hours   B. 2 hours   C. 8 hours
   D. 4 hours   E. 10 hours

9. Which of the following is NOT a great circle or part of a great circle?

   A. Arctic Circle
   B. 100th meridian
   C. Equator
   D. Shortest distance between New York and London
   E. Greenwich meridian

10. At which of the following places does the sun set EARLIEST on June 21?

    A. Montreal, Canada   B. Santiago, Chile
    C. Mexico City, Mexico   D. Lima, Peru
    E. Manila, P.I.

KEY (CORRECT ANSWERS)

TEST 1

1. C   5. A
2. E   6. B
3. C   7. B
4. A   8. C

TEST 2

1. C
2. B

TEST 3

1. B   6. D
2. A   7. D
3. C   8. E
4. C   9. C
5. D

TEST 4

1. A
2. B
3. C
4. C
5. D

TEST 5

1. D   5. D
2. B   6. E
3. A   7. A
4. E

TEST 6

1. E   5. B
2. A   6. B
3. C   7. B
4. D

TEST 7

1. A   6. C
2. A   7. E
3. D   8. D
4. C   9. E
5. D   10. E
          11. D

TEST 8

1. D   6. A
2. C   7. D
3. C   8. B
4. E   9. C
5. D   10. D

TEST 9

1. E   5. D
2. B   6. A
3. B   7. D
4. D

TEST 10

1. B   6. D
2. D   7. B
3. A   8. A
4. D   9. D
5. A   10. E

TEST 11

1. A   5. D
2. C   6. C
3. B   7. A
4. C

TEST 12

1. B   6. C
2. D   7. D
3. C   8. E
4. B   9. A
5. C   10. B

ARITHMETICAL COMPUTATION AND REASONING
EXAMINATION SECTION
TEST 1

DIRECTIONS: Each question or incomplete statement is followed by several suggested answers or completions. Select the one that BEST answers the question or completes the statement. *PRINT THE LETTER OF THE CORRECT ANSWER IN THE SPACE AT THE RIGHT.*

1. 3/8 less than $40 is 1.____
   A. $25 B. $65 C. $15 D. $55

2. 27/64 expressed as a percent is 2.____
   A. 40.625% B. 42.188% C. 43.750% D. 45.313%

3. 1/6 more than 36 gross is _____ gross. 3.____
   A. 6 B. 48 C. 30 D. 42

4. 15 is 20% of 4.____

5. The number which when increased by 1/3 of itself equals 96 is 5.____
   A. 128 B. 72 C. 64 D. 32

6. 0.16 3/4 written as percent is 6.____
   A. 16 3/4% B. 16.3/4% C. .016 3/4% D. .0016 3/4%

7. 55% of 15 is 7.____
   A. 82.5 B. 0.825 C. 0.0825 D. 8.25

8. The number which when decreased by 1/3 of itself equals 96 is 8.____
   A. 64 B. 32 C. 128 D. 144

9. A carpenter used a board 15 3/4 ft. long from which 3 footstools were made with sufficient lumber left over for half of another footstool. 9.____
   If the lumber cost 24 1/2¢ per foot, the cost of EACH footstool was
   A. $1.54 B. $3.86 C. $1.10 D. $1.08

10. In one year, a luncheonette purchased 1231 gallons of milk for $907.99. 10.____
    The AVERAGE cost per half pint was
    A. $0.046 B. $0.045 C. $0.047 D. $0.044

11. The product of 23 and 9 3/4 is 11.____
    A. 191 2/3 B. 224 1/4 C. 213 3/4 D. 32 3/4

12. An order for 345 machine bolts at $4.15 per hundred will cost 12.____
    A. $0.1432 B. $1.1432 C. $14.32 D. $143.20

13. The fractional equivalent of .0625 is

    A. 1/16   B. 1/15   C. 1/14   D. 1/13

14. The number 0.03125 equals

    A. 3/64   B. 1/16   C. 1/64   D. 1/32

15. 21.70 divided by 1.75 equals

    A. 124   B. 12.4   C. 1.24   D. .124

16. The average cost of school lunches for 100 children varied as follows: Monday, $0.285; Tuesday, $0.237; Wednesday, $0.264; Thursday, $0.276; Friday, $0.292. The AVERAGE lunch cost

    A. $0.136   B. $0.270   C. $0.135   D. $0.271

17. The cost of 5 dozen eggs at $8.52 per gross is

    A. $3.50   B. $42.60   C. $3.55   D. $3.74

18. 410.07 less 38.49 equals

    A. 372.58   B. 371.58   C. 381.58   D. 382.68

19. The cost of 7 3/4 tons of coal at $20.16 per ton is

    A. $15.12   B. $151.20   C. $141.12   D. $156.24

20. The sum of 90.79, 79.09, 97.90, and 9.97 is

    A. 277.75   B. 278.56   C. 276.94   D. 277.93

KEY (CORRECT ANSWERS)

1.	A	11.	B
2.	B	12.	C
3.	D	13.	A
4.	C	14.	D
5.	B	15.	B
6.	A	16.	D
7.	D	17.	C
8.	D	18.	B
9.	C	19.	D
10.	A	20.	A

SOLUTIONS TO PROBLEMS

1. ($40)(5/8) = $25

2. 27/64 = .421875 ≈ 42.188%

3. (36)(1 1/6) = 42

4. Let x = missing number. Then, 15 = .20x. Solving, x = 75

5. Let x = missing number. Then, x + 1/3 x = 96. Simplifying, 4/3 x = 96. Solving, x = 96 ÷ 4/3 = 72

6. .16 3/4 = 16 3/4% by simply moving the decimal point two places to the right.

7. (.55)(15) = 8.25

8. Let x = missing number. Then, x - 1/3 x = 96. Simplifying, 2/3 x = 96. Solving, x = 96 ÷ 2/3 = 144

9. 15 3/4 ÷ 3 1/2 = 4.5 feet per footstool. The cost of one footstool is ($.245)(4.5) = $1.1025 ≈ $1.10

10. $907.99 ÷ 1231 = $.7376 per gallon. Since there are 16 half-pints in a gallon, the average cost per half-pint is $.7376 ÷ 16 ≈ $.046

11. (23)(9 3/4) = (23)(9.75) = 224.25 or 224 1/4

12. ($4.15)(3.45) = $14.3175 = $14.32

13. .0625 = 625/10,000 = 1/16

14. .03125 = 3125/100,000 = 1/32

15. 21.70 ÷ 1.75 = 12.4

16. The sum of these lunches is $1.354. Then, $1.354 ÷ 5 = $.2708 = $.271

17. $8.52 ÷ 12 = $.71 per dozen. Then, the cost of 5 dozen is ($.71)(5) = $3.55

18. 410.07 - 38.49 = 371.58

19. ($20.16)(7.75) = $156.24

20. 90.79 + 79.09 + 97.90 + 9.97 = 277.75

TEST 2

DIRECTIONS: Each question or incomplete statement is followed by several suggested answers or completions. Select the one that BEST answers the question or completes the statement. *PRINT THE LETTER OF THE CORRECT ANSWER IN THE SPACE AT THE RIGHT.*

1. 1600 is 40% of what number? 1._____
   A. 6400   B. 3200   C. 4000   D. 5600

2. An executive's time card reads: Arrived 9:15 A.M., Left 2:05 P.M. 2._____
   How many hours was he in the office? _____ hours _____ minutes.
   A. 5; 10   B. 4; 50   C. 4; 10   D. 5; 50

3. .4266 times .3333 will have the following number of decimals in the product: 3._____
   A. 8   B. 4   C. 1   D. None of these

4. An office floor is 25 ft. wide by 36 ft. long. 4._____
   To cover this floor with carpet will require _____ square yards.
   A. 100   B. 300   C. 900   D. 25

5. 1/8 of 1% expressed as a decimal is 5._____
   A. .125   B. .0125   C. 1.25   D. .00125

6. $\dfrac{6 \div 4}{6 \times 4}$ equals 6x4 6._____
   A. 1/16   B. 1   C. 1/6   D. 1/4

7. 1/25 of 230 equals 7._____
   A. 92.0   B. 9.20   C. .920   D. 920

8. 4 times 3/8 equals 8._____
   A. 1 3/8   B. 3/32   C. 12.125   D. 1.5

9. 3/4 divided by 4 equals 9._____
   A. 3   B. 3/16   C. 16/3   D. 16

10. 6/7 divided by 2/7 equals 10._____
    A. 6   B. 12/49   C. 3   D. 21

11. The interest on $240 for 90 days ' 6% is 11._____
    A. $4.80   B. $3.40   C. $4.20   D. $3.60

12. 16 2/3% of 1728 is 12._____
    A. 91   B. 288   C. 282   D. 280

13. 6 1/4% of 6400 is   13.____
    A. 2500   B. 410   C. 108   D. 400

14. 12 1/2% of 560 is   14.____
    A. 65   B. 40   C. 50   D. 70

15. 2 yards divided by 3 equals   15.____
    A. 2 feet   B. 1/2 yard   C. 3 yards   D. 3 feet

16. A school has 540 pupils. 45% are boys. How many girls are there in this school?   16.____
    A. 243   B. 297   C. 493   D. 394

17. .1875 is equivalent to   17.____
    A. 18 3/4   B. 75/18   C. 18/75   D. 3/16

18. A kitchen cabinet listed at $42 is sold for $33.60. The discount allowed is   18.____
    A. 10%   B. 15%   C. 20%   D. 30%

19. 3 6/8 divided by 8 1/4 equals   19.____
    A. 9 1/8   B. 12   C. 5/11   D. 243.16

20. An agent sold goods to the amount of $1480. His commission at 5 1/2% was   20.____
    A. $37.50   B. $81.40   C. 76.70   D. $81.10

KEY (CORRECT ANSWERS

1. C   11. D
2. B   12. B
3. A   13. D
4. A   14. D
5. D   15. A

6. A   16. B
7. B   17. D
8. D   18. C
9. B   19. C
10. C   20. B

3 (#2)

SOLUTIONS TO PROBLEMS

1. Let x = missing number. Then, 1600 = .40x. Solving, x = 4000

2. 2:05 PM - 9:15 AM = 4 hours 50 minutes

3. The product of two 4-decimal numbers is an 8-decimal number.

4. (25 ft)(36 ft) = 900 sq.ft. = 100 sq.yds.

5. (1/8)(1%) = (.125)(.01) = .00125

6. (6 ÷ 4) ÷ (6 x 4) = 3/2 ÷ 24 = (3/2)(1/24) = (1/16)

7. (1/25)(230) = 9.20

8. (4)(3/8) = 12/8 = 1.5

9. 3/4 ÷ 4 = (3/4)(1/4) = 3/16

10. 6/7 / 2/7 = (6/7)(7/2) = 3

11. ($240)(.06)(90/360) = $3.60

12. (16 2/3%)(1728) = (1/6)(1728) = 288

13. (6 1/4%)(6400) = (1/16)(6400) = 400

14. (12 1/2%)(560) = (1/8)(560) = 70

15. 2 yds ÷ 3 = 2/3 yds = (2/3)(3) = 2 ft.

16. If 45% are boys, then 55% are girls. Thus, (540)(.55) = 297

17. .1875 = 1875/10,000 = 3/16

18. $42 - $33.60 = $8.40.
    The discount is $8.40 ÷ $42 = .20 = 20%

19. 3 6/8 - 8 1/4 = (30/8)(4/33) = 5/11

20. ($1480)(.055) = $81.40

TEST 3

DIRECTIONS: Each question or incomplete statement is followed by several suggested answers or completions. Select the one that BEST answers the question or completes the statement. *PRINT THE LETTER OF THE CORRECT ANSWER IN THE SPACE AT THE RIGHT.*

1. 93.648 divided by 0.4 is

    A. 23.412 B. 234.12 C. 2.3412 D. 2341.2

2. Add 4.3682, .0028, 34., 9.92, and from the sum subtract 1.992. The remainder is

    A. .46299 B. 4.6299 C. 462.99 D. 46.299

3. At $2.88 per gross, three dozen will cost

    A. $8.64 B. $0.96 C. $0.72 D. $11.52

4. 13 times 2.39 times 0.024 equals

    A. 745.68 B. 74.568 C. 7.4568 D. .74568

5. A living room suite is marked $64 less 25 percent. A cash discount of 10 percent is allowed.
   The cash price is

    A. $53.20 B. $47.80 C. $36.00 D. $43.20

6. 1/8 of 1 percent expressed as a decimal is

    A. .125 B. .0125 C. 1.25 D. .00125

7. 16 percent of 482.11 equals

    A. 77.1376 B. 771.4240 C. 7714.2400 D. 7.71424

8. A merchant sold a chair for $60. This was at a profit of 25 percent of what it cost him. The chair cost him

    A. $48 B. $45 C. $15 D. $75

9. Add 5 hours 13 minutes, 3 hours 49 minutes, and 14 minutes. The sum is _____ hours _____ minutes.

    A. 9; 16 B. 9; 76 C. 8; 16 D. 8; 6

10. 89 percent of $482 is

    A. $428.98 B. $472.36 C. $42.90 D. $47.24

11. 200 percent of 800 is

    A. 16 B. 1600 C. 2500 D. 4

12. Add 2 feet 3 inches, 4 feet 11 inches, 8 inches, 6 feet 6 inches. The sum is _____ feet _____ inches.

    A. 12; 4 B. 12; 14 C. 14; 4 D. 14; 28

13. A merchant bought dresses at $15 each and sold them at $20 each. His overhead expenses are 20 percent of cost. His net profit on each dress is   13.____

    A. $1   B. $2   C. $3   D. $4

14. 0.0325 expressed as a percent is   14.____

    A. 325%   B. 3 1/4%   C. 32 1/2%   D. 32.5%

15. Add 3/4, 1/8, 1/32, 1/2; and from the sum subtract 4/8. The remainder is   15.____

    A. 2/32   B. 7/8   C. 29/32   D. 3/4

16. A salesman gets a commission of 4 percent on his sales. If he wants his commission to amount to $40, he will have to sell merchandise totaling   16.____

    A. $160   B. $10   C. $1,000   D. $100

17. Jones borrowed $225,000 for five years at 3 1/2 percent. The annual interest charge was   17.____

    A. $1,575   B. $1,555   C. $7,875   D. $39,375

18. A kitchen cabinet listed at $42 is sold for $33.60. The discount allowed is _____ percent.   18.____

    A. 10   B. 15   C. 20   D. 30

19. The exact number of days from May 5, 2007 to July 1, 2007 is _____ days.   19.____

    A. 59   B. 58   C. 56   D. 57

20. A dealer sells an article at a loss of 50% of the cost. Based on the selling price, the loss is   20.____

    A. 25%   B. 50%   C. 100%   D. none of these

KEY (CORRECT ANSWERS)

1. B   11. B
2. D   12. C
3. C   13. B
4. D   14. B
5. D   15. C

6. D   16. C
7. A   17. C
8. A   18. C
9. A   19. D
10. A   20. C

SOLUTIONS TO PROBLEMS

1. 93.648 ÷ .4 = 234.12

2. 4.368 + .0028 + 34 + 9.92 - 1.992 = 48.291 - 1.992 = 46.299

3. $2.88 for 12 dozen means $.24 per dozen. Three dozen will cost (3)($.24) = $.72

4. (13)(2.39)(.024) = .74568

5. ($64)(.75)(.90) = $43.20

6. (1/8)(1%) = (.125)(.01) = .00125

7. (.16)(482.11) = 77.1376

8. Let x = cost. Then, 1.25x = $60. Solving, x = $48

9. 5 hrs. 13 min. + 3 hrs. 49 min. + 14 min = 8 hrs. 76 min.

10. (.89)($482) = $428.98

11. 200% = 2. So, (200%)(800) = (2)(800) = 1600

12. 2 ft. 3 in. + 4 ft. 11 in. + 8 in. + 6 ft. 6 in. + 12 ft. 28 in. = 14 ft. 4 in.

13. Overhead is (.20)($15) = $3. The net profit is $20 - $15 - $3 = $2

14. .0325 = 3.25% = 3 1/4%

15. 3/4 + 1/8 + 1/32 + 1/2 - 4/8 = 45/32 - 4/8 = 29/32

16. Let x = sales. Then, $40 = .04$x$. Solving, x = $1000

17. Annual interest is ($225,000)(.035) x 1 = 7875

18. $42 - $33.60 = $8.40. Then, $8.40 ÷ $42 = .20 = 20%

19. The number of days left for May, June, July is 26, 30, and 1. Thus, 26 + 30 + 1 = 57

20. Let x = cost, so that .50x = selling price. The loss is represented by .50x ÷ .50x = 1 = 100% on the selling price. (Note: The loss in dollars is x - .50x = .50x)

ARITHMETIC

EXAMINATION SECTION
TEST 1

DIRECTIONS: Each question or incomplete statement is followed by several suggested answers or completions. Select the one that BEST answers the question or completes the statement. *PRINT THE LETTER OF THE CORRECT ANSWER IN THE SPACE AT THE RIGHT.*

1. 215 x 30 =
   - A. 650
   - B. 6450
   - C. 6500
   - D. None of the above

   1.____

2. How much is saved by buying a $60 bicycle for cash instead of paying $5.25 a month for a year?
   - A. $3.00
   - B. $6.00
   - C. $7.50
   - D. None of the above

   2.____

3. How many square inches are in a square foot?
   - A. 12
   - B. 24
   - C. 144
   - D. None of the above

   3.____

4. What is ten thousand multiplied by one thousand?
   - A. One hundred thousand
   - B. One million
   - C. Ten million
   - D. None of the above

   4.____

5. 4 1/6 + 3 1/12 =
   - A. $7\frac{1}{4}$
   - B. $7\frac{7}{12}$
   - C. $8\frac{1}{4}$
   - D. None of the above

   5.____

6. Tom is awake an average of 15 hours each day. How many hours does he sleep in a week?
   - A. 9
   - B. 45
   - C. 105
   - D. None of the above

   6.____

7. If peppermints costing 70¢ per lb. come in 1 1/2 lb. boxes, what is the cost of 5 boxes?
   - A. $3.50
   - B. $5.25
   - C. $5.75
   - D. None of the above

   7.____

8. What is 349,638 rounded to the nearest hundred?
   - A. 349,600
   - B. 349,640
   - C. 350,000
   - D. None of the above

   8.____

9. 6 1/9 - 3 1/3 =

   A. 2 7/9
   B. 2 8/9
   C. 3 1/2
   D. None of the above

10. Which is less than one-thousandth of an inch?

    A. .025 in.
    B. .004 in.
    C. .0008 in.
    D. None of the above

11. Which is ten million three thousand?

    A. 10,300,000
    B. 10,030,000
    C. 10,003,000
    D. None of the above

12. $\frac{1}{2} + \frac{1}{3} + \frac{1}{6}$

    A. $\frac{1}{11}$
    B. $\frac{5}{6}$
    C. 1
    D. None of the above

13. 2/5 of 20 =

    A. 1/8
    B. 8
    C. 50
    D. None of the above

14. In the following multiplication, N stands for a number.

    4N5
    × 4
    ─────
    1740

    What is the number?

    A. 3
    B. 6
    C. 8
    D. None of the above

15. 7/8 - 1/2

    A. 3/8
    B. 3/4
    C. 1
    D. None of the above

16. The scale for a house plan is 1/4 in. =1 ft. How long is a hall that is 3 inches long on the plan?

    A. 7 ft.
    B. $12\frac{1}{2}$ ft.
    C. 16 ft.
    D. None of the above

17. 4 1/5 x 1 3/7 =

    A. 5
    B. 5 22/35
    C. 6
    D. None of the above

18. 7/3 - 11/6

   A. 1/2
   B. 1 3/11
   C. 1 1/3
   D. None of the above

18.____

19. The school pool is 60 feet long.
    How many lengths must John swim to pass his 100-yard swimming test?

   A. 2
   B. 5
   C. 6
   D. None of the above

19.____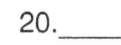

20. A store bought a dozen clocks for $72 and sold each for 50% more than it cost. What was the selling price of one clock?

   A. $6.50
   B. $9.00
   C. $26.00
   D. None of the above

20.____

21. If J stands for John's age and F for his father's age, which shows that John is 26 years younger than his father?

   A. J + F = 26
   B. J-26=F
   C. J + 26 = F
   D. None of the above

21.____

22. The board at the right has five equally spaced holes. What is the distance between the centers of holes 2 and 3?

   A. 8"
   B. 10"
   C. 20"
   D. None of the above

22.____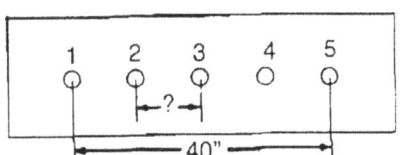

23. .07)51.1 =

   A. 7.3
   B. 73
   C. 730
   D. None of the above

23.____

24. Joe worked from 8:30 A.M. until 4:45 P.M., except for 45 minutes for lunch. How many hours did he work?

   A. $6\frac{1}{2}$
   B. $7\frac{1}{2}$
   C. $8\frac{1}{2}$
   D. None of the above

24.____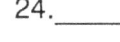

25. A highway 150 miles long cost $130 million. What was the AVERAGE cost per mile?

   A. Between $12,000 and $13,000
   B. Between $200,000 and $300,000
   C. Between $800,000 and $900,000
   D. None of the above

25.____

KEY (CORRECT ANSWERS)

1. B
2. A
3. C
4. C
5. A

6. D
7. B
8. A
9. A
10. C

11. C
12. C
13. B
14. A
15. A

16. D
17. C
18. A
19. B
20. B

21. C
22. B
23. C
24. B
25. C

SOLUTIONS TO PROBLEMS

1. $(215)(30) = 6450$

2. Savings = $(\$5.25)(12) - \$60 = \$3.00$

3. $(12)(12) = 144$ sq.in. = 1 sq.ft.

4. $(10,000)(1000) = 10,000,000 =$ ten million

5. $4\frac{1}{6} + 3\frac{1}{12} = 4\frac{2}{12} + 3\frac{1}{12} = 7\frac{3}{12} = 7\frac{1}{4}$

6. $(9)(7) = 63$ hours of sleep per week

7. $(5)(1\frac{1}{2})(.70) = \$5.25$

8. $349,638 = 349,600$ when rounded to the nearest hundred

9. $6\frac{1}{9} - 3\frac{1}{3} = 6\frac{1}{9} - 3\frac{3}{9} = 5\frac{10}{9} - 3\frac{3}{9} = 2\frac{7}{9}$

10. .0008 in. is less than .001 in.

11. $10,003,000 =$ ten million three thousand

12. $\frac{1}{2} + \frac{1}{3} + \frac{1}{6} = \frac{3}{6} + \frac{2}{6} + \frac{1}{6} = 1$

13. $(\frac{2}{5})(\frac{20}{1}) = \frac{40}{5} = 8$

14. If N = 3, we have $(435)(4) = 1740$. Note: $(5)(4) = 0$ digit and a carry-over of 2 in this multiplication. So, $4 \times N + 2 = 1$ digit Only N = 3 or N = 8 would fit. But note that the final answer of 1740 would eliminate 8 as a choice.

15. $\frac{7}{8} - \frac{1}{2} = \frac{7}{8} - \frac{4}{8} = \frac{3}{8}$

16. $3" \div \frac{1}{4} = 12$. Then, $(12)(1 \text{ ft.}) = 12$ ft.

17. $4\frac{1}{5} \times 1\frac{3}{7} = (\frac{21}{5})(\frac{10}{7}) = \frac{210}{35} = 6$

18. $\frac{7}{3} - \frac{11}{6} = \frac{14}{6} - \frac{11}{6} = \frac{3}{6} = \frac{1}{2}$

6 (#1)

19. 100 yds. = 300 ft. Then, 300 ÷ 60 = 5 lengths

20. $72 12 = $6.00. Then, ($6.00)(1.50) = $9.00

21. J + 26 = F shows that John is 26 years younger than his father.

22. The distance from hole 1 to hole 5 = 40", so the distance between any two consecutive holes = 40" ÷ 4 = 10"

23. 51.1 ÷ .07 = 730

24. From 8:30 AM to 4:45 PM = 8 8i hrs. Then, hrs. of 3 work. (Note: 45 min. = 3/4 hr.)

25. $130,000,000 ÷ 150 = = $866,666.67 average cost per mile.

   This figure is between $800,000 and $900,000.

———

TEST 2

DIRECTIONS: Each question or incomplete statement is followed by several suggested answers or completions. Select the one that BEST answers the question or completes the statement. *PRINT THE LETTER OF THE CORRECT ANSWER IN THE SPACE AT THE RIGHT.*

1. What is the volume of the box shown at the right?
    A. 7 cu. ft.
    B. 12 cu. ft.
    C. 14 cu. ft.
    D. None of the above

    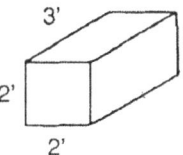

    1.____

2. If lemonade is made by mixing 1 pint of lemon juice with 3 quarts of water, how much lemon juice should be mixed with 3 gallons of water?

    A. 2 quarts
    B. 3 quarts
    C. 1 gallon
    D. None of the above

    2.____

3. What is the area of the figure shown at the right?
    A. 3 sq. in.
    B. 5 sq. in.
    C. 10 sq. in.
    D. None of the above

    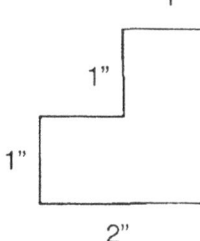

    3.____

4. $\dfrac{21 \times 14 \times 30}{28 \times 15 \times 7} =$

    A. 2
    B. 3
    C. 21
    D. None of the above

    4.____

5. 125% of 60 =

    A. 75
    B. 750
    C. 7500
    D. None of the above

    5.____

6. In the formula I = .05pt, I is the interest due on p dollars borrowed at 5% for t years. What is I if p = $500?

    A. 25t
    B. .10t
    C. .05(500+t)
    D. None of the above

    6.____

7. 4 x 6 = ? x 8. ? =

    A. 3
    B. 24
    C. 192
    D. None of the above

    7.____

8. On a day in January, the temperature in Central City was -18° F. How many degrees below freezing was this?

    A. 14
    B. 18
    C. 50
    D. None of the above

    8.____

9. .875 =

   A. $\dfrac{875}{100}$
   B. $\dfrac{5}{8}$
   C. 7 / 2
   D. None of the above

10. What is the area of the right triangle shown at the right?
    A. 6 sq. ft.
    B. 12 sq. ft.
    C. 60 sq. ft.
    D. None of the above

11. A United States Savings Bond costs $18.75. How many can be bought for $150?

    A. 6
    B. 8
    C. 12
    D. None of the above

12. One half of a melon was divided equally among 4 boys. What portion of the whole melon did each boy get?

    A. 1/8
    B. 1/6
    C. 1/4
    D. None of the above

13. One third of a foot is what part of a yard?

    A. 1/6
    B. 1/9
    C. 1/12
    D. None of the above

14. What is the sum of XXVIII and XII?

    A. D
    B. XC
    C. XL
    D. None of the above

15. How many people can each have pint of punch from one gallon of punch?

    A. 8
    B. 16
    C. 32
    D. None of the above

16. How much are license plates for a car weighing 3500 lbs. if the cost is $.50 per 100 lbs.?

    A. $17.50
    B. $35.00
    C. $70.00
    D. None of the above

17. What percent of the figure is black?

    A. 20%
    B. 25%
    C. 33 1/3%
    D. None of the above

18. Each week, Bill saves $2 of his own money and $3 given him by his father. When the total is $25, how much of it was from Bill's own money?

    A. $10.00
    B. $12.50
    C. $20.00
    D. None of the above

19. $\dfrac{3}{8} \div \dfrac{1}{4}$

    A. 25
    B. .5
    C. 1.5
    D. None of the above

19.____

20. If the price of a $5 tablecloth is reduced by $1, what is the percent reduction?

    A. 4%
    B. 20%
    C. 25%
    D. None of the above

20.____

KEY (CORRECT ANSWERS)

1. B
2. A
3. A
4. B
5. A
6. A
7. A
8. C
9. C
10. A
11. B
12. A
13. B
14. C
15. B
16. A
17. B
18. A
19. C
20. B

4 (#2)

SOLUTIONS TO PROBLEMS

1. Volume = (2')(2')(3') = 12 cu.ft.

2. 3 gallons = 12 qts. and 12 qts. 3 qts. = 4.
   Thus, (1 pt)(4) = 4 pts = 2 qts of lemon juice.

3. Area of I = 1" x 1" = 1 sq.in.
   Area of II = 2" x 1" = 2 sq.in.
   Total area = 3 sq.in.

4. [(21)(14)(30)] ÷ [(28)(15)(7)] = 8820 ÷ 2940 = 3

5. (1.25)(60) = 75

6. I = (.05)($500)(t) = 25t

7. 4 x 6 = 24. Then, 24 ÷ 8 = 3

8. $-18°F = 32° - (-18°) = 50°$ below freezing

9. $.875 = \dfrac{875}{1000} = \dfrac{7}{8}$

10. Area = (1/2)(3')(4') = 6 sq.ft.

11. $150 ÷ $18.75 = 8 bonds

12. $\dfrac{1}{2} \div 4 = \dfrac{1}{2} \times \dfrac{1}{4} = \dfrac{1}{8}$ melon

13. $\dfrac{1}{3} \text{ft} = (\dfrac{1}{3})(12") = 4"$ and $\dfrac{4"}{36"} = \dfrac{1}{9}$ yd.

14. XXVIII + XII = 28 + 12 = 40 = XL

15. 1 gallon = 8 pints. 8 Pints ÷ $\dfrac{1}{2}$ Pint = 16 servings

16. 3500 ÷ 100 = 35, so (35)($.50) = $17.50

17. $\dfrac{3}{12}$ = 25% of these boxes are black

18. Let x = Bill's own money. Then, $\dfrac{2}{5}=\dfrac{x}{25}$ Solving, x = $10

19. $\dfrac{3}{8}\div\dfrac{1}{4}=(\dfrac{3}{8})(\dfrac{4}{1})=\dfrac{12}{8}=1.5$

20. $\dfrac{1}{5}$ = 20% reduction

ARITHMETICAL REASONING
EXAMINATION SECTION
TEST 1

DIRECTIONS: Each question or incomplete statement is followed by several suggested answers or completions. Select the one that BEST answers the question or completes the statement. *PRINT THE LETTER OF THE CORRECT ANSWER IN THE SPACE AT THE RIGHT.*

1. The population of a city is, approximately, 7.85 million. The area is approximately 200 square miles. The number of thousand persons per square mile is
   A. 3.925   B. 39.25   C. 392.5   D. 39250

2. The longest straight line that can be drawn to connect two points on the circumference of a circle whose radius is 9 inches is
   A. 9 inches   B. 18 inches   C. 28.2753 inches   D. 4.5 inches

3. It is believed that every even number is the sum of two prime numbers. Two prime numbers whose sum is 32 are
   A. 7, 25   B. 22, 21   C. 13, 19   D. 17, 15

4. To divide a number by 3000, we should *move* the decimal point 3 places to the
   A. right and divide by 3
   B. left and divide by 3
   C. right and multiply by 3
   D. left and multiply by 3

5. The difference between the area of a rectangle 6 ft. by 4 ft. and the area of a square having the *same* perimeter is
   A. 1 sq. ft.   B. 2 sq. ft.   C. 4 sq. ft.   D. none of these

6. The ratio of 1/4 to 3/8 is the *same* as the ratio of
   A. 1 to 3   B. 2 to 3   C. 3 to 2   D. 3 to 4

7. If 7½ is divided by 1 1/5, the quotient is
   A. 6 1/4   B. 9   C. 7 1/10   D. 6 3/5

8. A farmer has a cylindrical metal tank for watering his stock. It is 10 ft. in diameter and 3 ft. deep. If one cubic foot contains about 7.5 gallons, the *approximate* capacity of the tank in gallons is
   A. 12   B. 225   C. 4   D. 1707

9. The fraction which fits in the following series, 1/2, 1/10, _____, 1/250, is
   A. 1/20   B. 1/100   C. 1/10   D. 1/50

10. In two years, $200 with interest compounded semi-annually at 4% will amount to
    A. $216.48   B. $233.92   C. $208   D. $216

2 (#1)

SOLUTIONS TO ARITHMETICAL REASONING

1. Answer: (B) 39.25

   $$\frac{40,000}{20)8,000,000}$$ (number of persons per square mile)(approximate population)

   Answer: 39.25 or (approximately) 40 (thousand persons per sq. mi.)

2. Answer: (B) 18 inches

   9" + 9" = 18 inches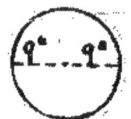

3. Answer: (C) 13, 19
   A prime number is an integer which cannot be divided by itself and one integer; a whole number as opposed to a fraction or a decimal.

4. Answer: (B) 3 places to the left and divide by

   $$\frac{2}{3)6,000.}$$

5. Answer: (A) 1 sq. ft.

   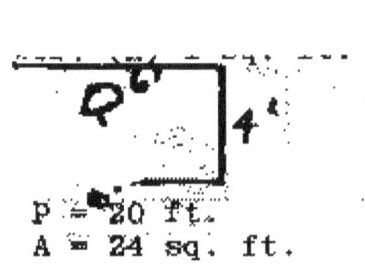
   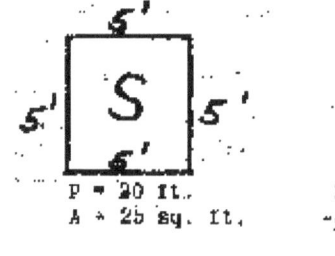

   P = 20 ft.   P = 20 ft.
   A = 24 sq.   A = 25 sq.

6. Answer: (B) 2 to 3

   $$\frac{1/4}{3/8} = 1/4 \div 3/8 = 1/4 \times 3/8 = 2/3$$

7. Answer: (A) 6 1/4

   $$\frac{7\ 1/2}{1\ 1/2} = \frac{15}{2} \div \frac{6}{5} = \frac{15}{2} \times \frac{5}{6} = \frac{25}{4} = 6\frac{1}{4} \quad \text{OR} \quad 1.2)\overline{7.5\ \tfrac{1}{4}} = 6\tfrac{3}{12}$$

3 (#1)

8. Answer: (B) 225

   $A = \pi R^2$
   $= 3(5)^2$
   $= 75$ sq. ft.

   225
   ×7.5
   ───
   1125
   1575   gal
   ───
   1687.5

   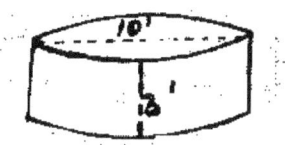

   Volume of tank = 75 × 3 = 225 cu. ft.
   (approximate capacity of tank in gallons)

9. Answer: (D) 1/50
   A geometric series: each number is multiplied by the same number to get the succeeding number. (Multiply each number by 1/5). ½, 1/10, 1/50/$216, 1/250. The missing number if 1/50.

10 Answer: (A) $216.48
    <u>Compound Interest</u>
    4% a year compounded semi-annually is the same as 2% for a half year

    A. $200 $200
       ×.02   × 4
       ─────   ─────
       $4.00 Interest for 1st half yr. $204 Principal for 1st half yr.

    B. $204 $204.00
       ×.02   × 4.08
       ─────   ──────
       $4.08 Interest for 2nd half yr. $208.08 Principal for 1st half of 2nd yr.

    C. $208.08 $208.08
       ×.02   × 4.16
       ──────   ──────
       $4.1616 Interest for 1st half of 2nd yr. $212.24 Principal for 2nd half of 2nd yr.

    D. $212.24 $212.24
       ×.02   × 4.24
       ──────   ──────
       $4.2448 Interest for 2nd half of 2nd yr. $216.48 Principal at end of 2nd half of 2nd yr.

TEST 2

DIRECTIONS: Each question or incomplete statement is followed by several suggested answers or completions. Select the one that BEST answers the question or completes the statement. *PRINT THE LETTER OF THE CORRECT ANSWER IN THE SPACE AT THE RIGHT.*

1. With a *tax rate* of .0200, a tax bill of $1050 corresponds to an *assessed valuation* of
   A. $21,000　　B. $52,500　　C. $21　　D. $1029

   1.____

2. A sales agent, after deducting his commission of 6%, remits $2491 to his principal. The SALE amounted to
   A. $2809　　B. $2640　　C. $2650　　D. $2341.54

   2.____

3. The percent equivalent of .0295 is
   A. 2.95%　　B. 29.5%　　C. .295%　　D. 295%

   3.____

4. An angle of 105 degrees is a _____ angle.
   A. straight　　B. acute　　C. obtuse　　D. reflex

   4.____

5. A quart is approximately sixty cubic inches. A cu. ft. of water weighs approximately sixty pounds. Therefore, a quart of water weights *approximately*
   A. 2 lbs.　　B. 3 lbs.　　C. 4 lbs.　　D. 5 lbs.

   5.____

6. If the *same* number is added to both the numerator and the denominator of a proper fraction, the
   A. value of the fraction is decreased
   B. value of the fraction is increased
   C. value of the fraction is unchanged
   D. effect of the operation depends on the original fraction

   6.____

7. The *lease common multiple* of 3, 8, 9, 12 is
   A. 36　　B. 72　　C. 108　　D. 144

   7.____

8. On a bill of $100, the *difference* between a discount of 30% and 20% and a discount of 40% and 10% is
   A. nothing　　B. $2　　C. $20　　D. 20%

   8.____

9. 1/3 percent of a number is 24. The NUMBER is
   A. 8　　B. 72　　C. 800　　D. 7200

   9.____

10. The cost of importing five dozen china dinner sets, billed at $32 per set, and paying a duty of 40% is
    A. $224　　B. $2688　　C. $768　　D. $1344

    10.____

SOLUTIONS TO ARITHMETICAL REASONING

1. Answer: (B) $52,500
   0200x = $1050   2x = $105,000
   200x = $10,500,000   x = $52,500 (assessed valuation)

2. Answer: (C) $2650
   $2491 + .06x = x
   x = 2491 + .06x

   |Proof|
   |$2650 $2491|
   |× .06   + 159|
   |$159.00 $2650|

   1.00x - .06x = 2491

   .94x = 2491
   .94x = 249,100

   $2,650
   94)249,100

3. Answer: (A) 2.95% [.0295 = 2.95%)

4. Answer: (C) obtuse angle
   An obtuse angle is an angle greater than 90°.

5. Answer: (A) 2 lbs.
   A quart = 60 cu. in.
   60 lbs. = 1 cu. ft. (or 1728 cu. in.) (12×12×12)
              (Keep like units of measure together)
   60 lbs. = 1728 cu. in.
   1 lb.   = 1728/60 = approximately .29 cu. in.
   If 29 cu. in. weighs 1 lb., then 60 cu. in. weighs 2 lbs. (approximately). Therefore, a quart weighs 2 lbs. (approximately).

6. Answer: (B) the value of the fraction is increased

   (1) Start with the fraction 2/3

   (2) $\frac{2+2}{3+2} = \frac{4}{5}$ (Adding 2 to the numerator and the denominator)

   (3) $\frac{3}{2} = \frac{10}{15}$

   (4) $\frac{4}{5} = \frac{12}{15}$

7. Answer: (B) 72
   Common multiple can be evenly divided by all the numbers. Lease common multiple: the lowest of these numbers.

3 (#2)

8. Answer: (B) $2
   Formula: Step 1. Express percentages as decimals
              Step 2. Subtract each discount from *one*
              Step 3. Multiply all the results
              Step 4. Subtract the product from *one*

   Step 1. .3, .2 and .4, .1
   Step 2. .7, .8 and .6, .9
   Step 3. .7 × .8 = .56 (represents percent remaining after the discounts
           .6 × .9 = .54   are taken)
   Step 4. 1.00   1.00
            -.56   -.54
             .44   .46

   Then, $100 × .02 = $2.00

9. Answer: (D) 7200

   $\frac{1}{300}x = 24;$ $x = 24 \times 300;$ $x = 7200$

10. Answer: (B) $2688

    $32
    ×60
    $1920   Cost of dinner sets before paying duty

    $1920
    ×.40
    $768.00   Duty

    $1920
    + 768
    $2688   Cost of dinner sets *after* paying duty

TEST 3

DIRECTIONS: Each question or incomplete statement is followed by several suggested answers or completions. Select the one that BEST answers the question or completes the statement. *PRINT THE LETTER OF THE CORRECT ANSWER IN THE SPACE AT THE RIGHT.*

1. A motorist travels 120 miles to his destination at the average speed of 60 miles per hour and returns to the starting point at the average speed of 40 miles per hour. His *average speed* for the ENTIRE trip is _____ miles per hour.
   A. 53   B. 50   C. 48   D. 45

2. A snapshot measures 2 1/2 inches by 1 7/8 inches. It is to be enlarged so that the longer dimension will be 4 inches. The length of the enlarged *shorter* dimension will be
   A. 2 1/2 inches   B. 3 3/8 inches   C. 3 inches   D. none of these

3. The approximate distance is, in feet, that an object falls in t seconds when dropped from a height is obtained by use of the formula $s = 16t^2$. In 8 seconds, the object will fall
   A. 15,384 feet   B. 1,024 feet   C. 256 feet   D. none of these

4. The PRODUCT of 75^3 and 75^7 is
   A. $(75)^{10}$ B. $(75)^{21}$ C. $(5,625)^{10}$ D. $(150)^{10}$

5. The scale of a map is: 3/4 of an inch = 10 miles. If the distance on the map between two towns is 6 inches, the *actual* distance is
   A. 45 miles   B. 60 miles   C. 80 miles   D. none of these

6. If $d = m \dfrac{50}{m}$, and m is a positive number which increases in value, d
   A. increases in value   B. decreases in value
   B. remains unchanged   D. fluctuates up and down in value

7. From a piece of tin in the shape of a square 6 inches on a side, the largest possible circle is cut out.
   Of the following, the ratio of the area of the circle to the area of the original square is *closest* in value to
   A. 4/5   B. 3/5   C. 2/3   D. 1/2

8. A pound of water is evaporated from 6 pounds of sea water containing 4% salt. The percentage of salt in the *remaining* solution is
   A. 3 1/3   B. 4   C. 4 4/5   D. none of these

9. If a cubic inch of a metal weighs 2 pounds, a cubic foot of the *same* metal weighs
   A. 8 pounds   B. 24 pounds   C. 288 pounds   D. none of these

10. Assume that, according to the Federal income tax law, if the taxable income in the case of a separate return is over $4,000, but not over $6,000, the tax is $840 + 26% of the excess over $4,000.
    If a taxpayer files a separate tax return and his taxable income is $5,500, the tax is

    A. $690   B. $1,230   C. $1,370   D. none of these

SOLUTIONS TO ARITHMETICAL REASONING

1. Answer: (C) 48 miles per hour
   120 miles = 2 hours (60 mph)
   120 miles = 3 hours (40 mph)
   240 miles = 5 hours = average of 48 mph

2. Answer: (C) 3 inches
   Change 2 1/2 to 20/8 Change 1 7/8 to 15/8
   Ratio is 20 to 15 or 4 to 3.
   If the longer dimension is 4 inches, then the shorter is 3 inches.

3. Answer: (B) 1,024 feet
   $s = 16 \times 8^2$ or 16×64 or 1024 feet

4. Answer: (A) $(75)^{10}$
   Because the 75 is constant, one needs only to add the exponents (7 and 3). Therefore, the product is 75^{10}.

5. Answer: (C) 80 miles
   $6 \div 3/4 = 6 \times 4/3 = 24/3$ or 8
   8×10 miles = 80 miles

6. Answer: (A) increases in value
   By increasing the value of my (by substituting numbers for letters), it is obvious that d increases in value.

7. Answer: (A) 4/5
   Area of square = 36 square inches
   Area of circle = π^2
   $\qquad = \pi 9 (3 \times 3)$
   $\qquad = 3\ 1/7 \times 9$
   $\qquad = 28\ 2/7$

   $$\frac{28\ 2/7}{36} = \frac{198}{7} \times \frac{1}{36} = \frac{198}{252}$$

   ```
           .78 = 78%
   252)198.00
       176 4
        21 60
        20 16
         1 44
   ```

   78% is closest to 4/5 (80%)

4 (#3)

8. Answer: (C) 4 4/5
.04 × 6 = .24 lbs. of salt in 6 lbs. of salt water
When a pound of water is evaporated, the salt content remains the same.

```
    .24
  5).24
   .04  4/5 = 4 4/5%
```

9. Answer: (D) none of these
1728 cubic inches   = 1 cubic foot
1 cubic inch   = 2 pounds
1728 cubic inches   = 3,456 pounds

10. Answer: (B) $1,230

$5,500
-4,000
$1,500 (excess over 4000)

$1500 × 25% = $390.00
              +840.00
              $1230.00 (tax)

TEST 4

DIRECTIONS: Each question or incomplete statement is followed by several suggested answers or completions. Select the one that BEST answers the question or completes the statement. *PRINT THE LETTER OF THE CORRECT ANSWER IN THE SPACE AT THE RIGHT.*

1. If the number of square inches in the area of a circle is equal to the number of inches in its circumference, the DIAMETER of the circle is   1.____
   A. 4 inches   B. 3 inches   C. 1 inch   D. none of these

2. The *least common multiple* of 20, 24, 32 is   2.____
   A. 900   B. 1,920   C. 15,360   D. none of these

3. Six quarts of a 20% solution of alcohol in water are mixed with 4 quarts of a 60% solution of alcohol in water. The *alcoholic* strength of the mixture is   3.____
   A. 80%   B. 50%   C. 36%   D. none of these

4. To find the radius of a circle whose circumference is 60 inches,   4.____
   A. multiply 60 by π
   B. divide 60 by 2π
   C. divide 30 by 2π
   D. divide 60 by π and extract the square root of the result

5. A micromillimeter is defined as one millionth of a millimeter. A length of 17 micromillimeters may be represented by   5.____
   A. .00017 mm.   B. 0000017 mm.
   C. .000017 mm.   D. .00000017 mm.

6. If 9x + 5 = 23, the numerical value of 18x + 5 is   6.____
   A. 46   B. 41   C. 32   D. 23 + 9x

7. When the fractions 2/3, 5/7, 8/11 and 9/13 are arranged in ascending order of size, the result is   7.____
   A. 8/11, 5/7, 9/13, 2/3   B. 5/7, 8/11, 2/3, 9/13
   C. 2/3, 8/11, 5/7, 9/13   D. 2/3, 9/13, 5/7, 8/11

8. If the outer diameter of a metal pipe is 2.84 inches and the inner diameter is 1.94 inches, the *thickness* of the metal is   8.____
   A. .45 of an inch   B. .90 of an inch   C. 1.94 inches   D. 2.39 inches

9. An office manager employs 3 typists at $450 per week, 2 general clerks at $400 per week, and a messenger at $320 per week. The *average* weekly wage of these part-time employees is   9.____
   A. $372.50   B. $390.00   C. $411.70   D. none of these

10. A rectangular bin 4 feet long, 3 feet wide, and 2 feet high is solidly packed with bricks whose dimensions are 8 inches, 4 inches, and 2 inches. The *number* of bricks in the bin is   10.____
    A. 54   B. 648   C. 1,298   D. none of these

SOLUTIONS TO ARITHMETICAL REASONING

1. Answer: (A) 4 inches
   Assume there are 100 square inches in the area of a circle and 100 inches in its circumference.
   A = 1/2Cr
   100 = 1/2 × Xr
   50r = 100
   r = 2
   d = 4

2. Answer: (D) none of these
   2)20 – 24 - 32
   2)10 – 12 – 16
   2)20 – 24 – 32
      5 – 3 – 4

   2 × 2 × 2 × 5 × 3 × 4 = 480

3. Answer: (C) 36%
   6 quarts × 20% = 120%
   4 quarts × 60% = 240%
   10 quarts   = 360%
   1 quart   = 36%

4. Answer: (B) divide 60 by 2

   C = 2r $r = \frac{60}{\pi} \times \frac{1}{2}$

   $2\pi r = 60$ $r = \frac{60}{2\pi}$

   $2r = \frac{60}{\pi}$

5. Answer: (C) .000017 mm.
   1 micromillimeter   =   .000001 mm.
   17 micromillimeters =   .000017 mm.

6. Answer: (B) 41
   9x + 5 = 23
   9x = 23 – 5 or 9x = 18
   x = 2
   18x + 5 = 36 + 5 or 41

7. Answer: (D) 2/3, 9/13, 5/7, 8/11
   Find the least common denominator = 3003

   $\frac{2}{3} = \frac{2002}{3003}$ $\frac{9}{13} = \frac{2079}{3003}$ $\frac{5}{7} = \frac{2145}{3003}$ $\frac{8}{11} = \frac{2184}{3003}$

   Correct order is 2/3, 9/13, 5/7, 8/11

8. Answer: (A) .45 of an inch
    2.84 inches = outer diameter
    1.94 inches = inner diameter
    .90 inches = thickness (both sides)
    .45 inches = thickness (one side)

9. Answer: (C) $41.17
    3 × 45 = $135
    2 × 40 = 80

    $\frac{1}{6}$ × 32 = $\frac{32}{\$247}$

    $247 ÷ 6 = $41 1/6 or $41.17

10. Answer: (B) 648

    There are 1728 cu. inches in 1 cu. ft. (12 × 12 × 12)
    4 × 3 × 2 = 24 cu.ft. × 1728 = 41472 cu. in. ÷ 64 (8 × 4 × 2) = 648 bricks

TEST 5

DIRECTIONS: Each question or incomplete statement is followed by several suggested answers or completions. Select the one that BEST answers the question or completes the statement. *PRINT THE LETTER OF THE CORRECT ANSWER IN THE SPACE AT THE RIGHT.*

1. If x is less than 10, and y is less than 5, it follows that
   A. x is greater than y
   B. x = 2y
   C. x-y = 5
   D. x+y is less than 15

2. A dealer sells an article at a loss of 50% of the cost. Based on the selling price, the *loss* is
   A. 25%
   B. 50%
   C. 100%
   D. none of these

3. If 8 men get together at a reunion and each man shakes hands once with each of the others, the *total number* of handshakes is
   A. 49
   B. 56
   C. 64
   D. 28

4. The world record for cycling a stretch of 20 kilometers is 26 minutes. This corresponds to an average speed of, *approximately*,
   A. 29 miles per hour
   B. 46 miles per hour
   C. 32 miles per hour
   D. none of these

5. The sum, s, of n consecutive integers beginning with 1 can be found by use of the formula $s = \frac{n(n+1)}{2}$. The sum of the *first 100 consecutive integers* is
   A. 5,001
   B. 5,050
   C. 10,000
   D. 10,100

6. Of the following, the value of $\frac{\sqrt[3]{64.32}}{\sqrt{.041}}$ is closest to
   A. 400
   B. 200
   C. 20
   D. 16

7. If each edge of a cube is increased by 2 inches, the
   A. volume is increased by 8 cubic inches
   B. area of each face is increased by 4 square inches
   C. diagonal of each face is increased by 2 inches
   D. sum of the edges is increased by 24 inches

8. In a school in which 40% of the enrolled students are boys, 80% of the boys are present on a certain day. If 1,152 boys are present, the total school enrollment is
   A. 1,440
   B. 2,880
   C. 3,600
   D. none of these

2 (#5)

9. An agent received a commission of d% of the selling price of a house. If the commission amounted to $600, the selling price, in dollars, was

    A. $\dfrac{60,000}{d}$ B. 600/d   C. 6d   D. 600d

9._____

10. A ship sails due north from a position 5 28' South Latitude to a position 6 43' North Latitude. Given that one minute of latitude is equivalent to 1 nautical mile, the ship has sailed a distance of _____ nautical miles
    A. 75   B. 371   C. 731   D. 1,211

10._____

SOLUTIONS TO ARITHMETICAL REASONING

1. Answer: (D) x + y is less than 15
   If x is less than 10 and y is less than 5, then x + y *MUST* be less than 15. None of the others is possible.

2. Answer: (C) 100%
   Based on selling price, the formula is written:
   Cost – Loss = Selling Price
   100% - 50% = 50%
   Loss = 100% of the Selling Price (loss equal to Selling Price)

3. Answer: (D) 28
   A shakes hands with the other 7
   B shakes hands with the other 6 (has already shaken A's)
   and so on……. Thus 7, 6, 5, 4, 3, 2, 1 = 28 handshakes

4. Answer: (A) 29 miles per hour
   1 kilometer = 5/8 of a mile
   20 kilometers = 20 × 5/8 = 12 1/2 miles
   12 1/2 miles : 26 minutes = x : 60 minutes
   26x = 750
   x = 28+ or 29 miles per hour

5. Answer: (B) 5,050

   $s = \dfrac{n(n+1)}{2}$ $s = \dfrac{100(100+1)}{2}$ $s = \dfrac{10,100}{2}$ $s = 5,050$

6. Answer: (C) 2

   $\sqrt[3]{64.32} = 4.01$ $\dfrac{4}{.2} = 4 \times \dfrac{10}{2} = 20$

   $\sqrt[2]{.041} = .202$

7. Answer: (D) the sum of the edges is increased by 24 inches. Since there are 12 edges to a cube and each edge is increased by 2 inches, the total increase is 24 inches.

8. Answer: (C) 3,600

   $1152 \div \dfrac{8}{10} = 1440 = 1440$ boys enrolled ($1152 \times 10/8$)

   $1440 \div \dfrac{4}{10} = 1440 \times \dfrac{10}{4}$ (total school enrollment)

9. Answer: (A) $\dfrac{60,000}{d}$

4 (#5)

$$600 \div d = 600 \times \frac{100}{d} = \frac{60{,}000}{d}$$

10. Answer: (C) 731 nautical miles

    5° 28'   1° = 60'
    6° 43'   11° = 660'
  11° 71'   + 71'
                                               731'

1' = 1 nautical mile
731' = 731 nautical miles

EXAMINATION SECTION
TEST 1

DIRECTIONS: Each question or incomplete statement is followed by several suggested answers or completions. Select the one that BEST answers the question or completes the statement. *PRINT THE LETTER OF THE CORRECT ANSWER IN THE SPACE AT THE RIGHT.*

Questions 1-10.

DIRECTIONS: In answering Questions 1 through 10, select the alternative that means the *same as* or the *opposite* of the word in italics.

1. *acquire*
   A. judge
   B. identify
   C. surrender
   D. educate
   E. happen

2. *begrudge*
   A. envy
   B. hate
   C. annoy
   D. obstruct
   E. punish

3. *obsolete*
   A. fatal
   B. modern
   C. distracting
   D. untouched
   E. broken

4. *inflexible*
   A. weak
   B. righteous
   C. harmless
   D. unyielding
   E. secret

5. *nominal*
   A. just
   B. slight
   C. cheerful
   D. familiar
   E. ceaseless

6. *debt*
   A. insane
   B. artificial
   C. skillful
   D. determined
   E. humble

7. *censure*
   A. focus
   B. exclude
   C. baffle
   D. portray
   E. praise

8. *nebulous*
   A. imaginary
   B. spiritual
   C. distinct
   D. starry-eyed
   E. unanswerable

9. *impart*
   A. hasten
   B. adjust
   C. gamble
   D. address
   E. communicate

10. *terminate*
    A. gain B. graduate C. harvest
    D. start E. paralyze

Questions 11-20.

DIRECTIONS: In answering Questions 11 through 20, select the word which, if inserted in the blank space, agrees MOST closely with the thought of the sentence.

11. Every good story is carefully contrived; the elements of the story are _____ to fi with one another in order to make an effect on the reader.
    A. read B. learned C. emphasized
    D. reduced E. planned

12. Their work was commemorative in character and consisted largely of _____ erected upon the occasion of victories.
    A. towers B. tombs C. monuments
    D. castles E. fortresses

13. Before criticizing the work of an artist, one needs to _____ the artist's purpose.
    A. understand B. reveal C. defend
    D. correct E. change

14. Because in the administration it hath respect not to the group but to the _____, our form of government is called a democracy.
    A. courts B. people C. majority
    D. individual E. law

15. Deductive reasoning is that form of reasoning in which the conclusion must necessarily follow if we accept the premise as true. In deduction, it is _____ for the premise to be true and the conclusion false.
    A. impossible B. inevitable C. reasonable
    D. surprising E. unlikely

16. Mathematics is the product of thought operating by means of _____ for the purpose of expressing general laws.
    A. reasoning B. symbols C. words
    D. examples E. science

17. No other man loss so much, so _____, so absolutely, as the beaten candidate for high public office.
    A. bewilderingly B. predictably C. disgracefully
    D. publicly E. cheerfully

18. Many television watchers enjoy stories which contain violence. Consequently, those television producers who are dominated by rating systems aim to _____ the popular taste.
    A. raise   B. control   C. gratify
    D. ignore   e. lower

    18.____

19. The latent period for the contractile response to direct stimulation of the muscle has quite another and shorter value, encompassing only a utilization period. Hence, it is that the term *latent period* must be _____ carefully each time that it is used.
    A. checked   B. timed   C. introduced
    D. defined   E. selected

    19.____

20. A man who cannot win honor in his own _____ will have a very small chance of winning it from posterity.
    A. right   B. field   C. country
    D. way   E. age

    20.____

Questions 21-35.

DIRECTIONS: In answering Questions 21 through 35, select the word that BEST completes the analogy.

21. Albino is to color as traitor is to
    A. patriotism   B. treachery   C. socialism
    D. integration   E. liberalism

    21.____

22. Senile is to infantile as supper is to
    A. snack   B. breakfast   C. dinner
    D. daytime   E. evening

    22.____

23. Snow shovel is to sidewalk as eraser is to
    A. writing   B. pencil   C. paper
    D. desk   E. mistake

    23.____

24. Lawyer is to court as soldier is to
    A. battle   B. victory   C. training
    D. rifle   E. discipline

    24.____

25. Faucet is to water as mosquito is to
    A. swamp   B. butterfly   C. cistern
    D. pond   E. malaria

    25.____

26. Astronomy is to geology as steeplejack is to
    A. mailman   B. surgeon   C. pilot
    D. miner   E. skindiver

    26.____

27. Chimney is to smoke as guide is to
    A. snare   B. compass   C. hunter
    D. firewood   E. wild game

28. Prodigy is to ability as ocean is to
    A. water   B. waves   C. ships
    D. icebergs   E. current

29. War is to devastation as microbe is to
    A. peace   B. flea   C. dog
    D. germ   E. pestilence

30. Blueberry is to pea a sky is to
    A. storm   B. world   C. star
    D. grass   E. purity

31. Pour is to spill as lie is to
    A. deception   B. misstatement   C. falsehood
    D. perjury   E. fraud

32. Disparage is to despise as praise is to
    A. dislike   B. adore   C. acclaim
    D. advocate   E. compliment

33. Wall is to mortar as nation is to
    A. family   B. people   C. patriotism
    D. geography   E. boundaries

34. Servant is to butter as pain is to
    A. cramp   B. hurt   C. illness
    D. itch   E. anesthesia

35. Fan is to air as newspaper is to
    A. literature   B. reporter   C. information
    D. subscription   E. reader

36. A set of papers is arranged and numbered from 1 to 49. If the paper numbered 3 is drawn first and every ninth paper thereafter, what will be the number of the last paper drawn?
    A. 45   B. 46   C. 47   D. 48   E. 49

37. Which quantity can be measured *exactly* from a tank of water by using only a 10-pint can and an 8-pint can? _____ pint(s)
    A. 1   B. 6   C. 3   D. 7   E. 5

38. If city R has more fires than city S, and city T has more fires than cities P and S combined, then the number of fires in city
    A. P must be less than in city T
    B. T must be less than in city R
    C. T must be greater than in city R
    D. R must be greater than in city P
    E. S must be greater than in city T

    38.____

39. The average of three numbers is 25.
    If one of the numbers is increased by 4, the average will remain unchanged if each of the other two numbers is reduced by
    A. 1   B. 2   C. 2/3   D. 4   E. 1 1/3

    39.____

40.
```
                    1
                 1     1
              1    2     1
           1    3     3    1
        1    4     6    4     1
     1     5    10    X     5     1
```
    Above are the first six rows of a triangular array constructed according to a fixed law.
    What number does the letter X represent?
    A. 8   B. 10   C. 15   D. 20   E. 5

    42.____

41. If all A are C and no C are B, it necessarily follows that
    A. all B are C   B. all B are A   C. no A are B
    D. no C are A   E. some B are A

    41.____

42. What number is missing in the series 7, ____, 63, 189?
    A. 9   B. 11   C. 19   D. 21   E. 24

    42.____

43. A clock that gains one minute each hour is synchronized at noon with a clock that loses two minutes an hour.
    How many minutes apart will the minute hands of the two clocks be at midnight?
    A. 0   B. 12   C. 14   D. 24   E. 30

    43.____

44. The pages of a typewritten report are numbered by hand from 1 to 100.
    How many times will it be necessary to write the numeral 5?
    A. 10   B. 11   C. 12   D. 19   E. 20

    44.____

45. The number 6 is called a *perfect* number because it is the sum of all its integral divisors except itself.
    Another *perfect* number is
    A. 12   B. 16   C. 24   D. 28   E. 36

    45.____

KEY (CORRECT ANSWERS)

1. C	11. E	21. A	31. B	41. C
2. A	12. C	22. B	32. B	42. D
3. B	13. A	23. C	33. C	43. D
4. D	14. D	24. A	34. A	44. E
5. B	15. A	25. E	35. C	45. D
6. C	16. B	26. D	36. D	
7. E	17. D	27. C	37. B	
8. C	18. C	28. A	38. A	
9. E	19. D	29. E	39. B	
10. D	20. E	30. D	40. B	

EXAMINATION SECTION
TEST 1

DIRECTIONS: In the space provided at the right, write the letter of the word or expression that most nearly expresses the meaning of the word printed in italics.

1. *Calligraphy* 1._____

    A. weaving
    B. handwriting
    C. drafting
    D. mapmaking

2. *Synchronize* 2._____

    A. happen at the same time
    B. follow immediately in time
    C. alternate between events
    D. postpone to a future time

3. *Semblance* 3._____

    A. surface
    B. diplomacy
    C. replacement
    D. appearance

4. *Circuitous* 4._____

    A. winding
    B. mutual
    C. exciting
    D. rugged

5. *Curtail* 5._____

    A. threaten
    B. strengthen
    C. lessen
    D. hasten

6. *Noxious* 6._____

    A. spicy
    B. smelly
    C. foreign
    D. harmful

7. *Drivel* 7._____

    A. fatigue
    B. scarcity
    C. nonsense
    D. waste

8. *Assuage* 8._____

    A. soothe
    B. cleanse
    C. enjoy
    D. reward

9. *Intrepid* 9._____

    A. exhausted
    B. fearless
    C. anxious
    D. youthful

10. *Treacherous* 10._____

    A. ignorant
    B. envious
    C. disloyal
    D. cowardly

11. The court jester served the role of *buffoon*

    A. horseman B. servant
    C. philosopher D. clown

12. The guest of honor began to speak *nonchalantly* to the audience.

    A. casually B. nervously
    C. seriously D. quietly

13. The governor gave the reporter a *terse* answer to the complex question.

    A. rambling B. inadequate
    C. brief D. ridiculous

14. The servants were told to *adorn* the statues.

    A. decorate B. remove
    C. wash D. destroy

15. Any further discussion of the problem would be *redundant*.

    A. unprofitable B. repetitive
    C. confusing D. misleading

16. The challenge to society is to prevent a criminal from operating with *impunity*.

    A. threats of violence
    B. lack of detection
    C. guarantees of success
    D. freedom from punishment

17. The politician's *candor* surprised his listeners.

    A. honesty B. comments
    C. viewpoint D. examples

18. The horror film was filled with zombies and *cadavers*.

    A. ghosts B. skeletons
    C. monsters D. corpses

19. Leslie worked *diligently* on her school project.

    A. skillfully B. resentfully
    C. industriously D. hurriedly

20. The supervisor could not *coerce* the employee to take early retirement.

    A. request B. force
    C. permit D. advise

21. *Stow*

    A. pack B. report
    C. interest D. beg

22. *Irrepressible*

    A. unrestrainable B. impatient
    C. unknowable D. impractical

23. *Grimace*

    A. important development B. point of view
    C. expression of disgust D. act of spite

24. *Promenade*

    A. limp B. walk
    C. jog   D. race

25. *Indicative*

    A. defensive   B. attractive
    C. disruptive D. suggestive

26. *Medley*

    A. game   B. entertainment
    C. discussion D. mixture

27. *Jaunty*

    A. mighty B. dirty
    C. lively D. petty

28. *Undue*

    A. genuine   B. wavy
    C. faultless D. inappropriate

29. *Visage*

    A. appearance B. vividness
    C. prospect   D. valor

30. *Avid*

    A. eager B. easy
    C. dry   D. flat

31. That *bestial* act marked him for life.

    A. unkind B. insensitive
    C. brutal D. spiteful

32. The professor was regarded as an *erudite* teacher.

    A. rigid   B. scholarly
    C. demanding D. reasonable

33. We could see the *knolls* from our window.

    A. rounded hills B. groups of trees
    C. high waves   D. marshes

34. As the nurse prepared the shot, I *winced* in anticipation.

    A. moaned aloud B. stared ahead
    C. lay still   D. shrank back

35. The president said that he would not *countenance* such policies.

    A. order
    B. implement
    C. approve
    D. introduce

36. The lawyer proved that the witness was a *prevaricator*.

    A. murderer
    B. liar
    C. thief
    D. fraud

37. The explorers followed the *tributary* to its origin.

    A. stream
    B. lake
    C. trail
    D. valley

38. She always comes to school *impeccably* groomed.

    A. carelessly
    B. conservatively
    C. stylishly
    D. flawlessly

39. Mrs. Royce *discreetly* answered all the questions asked about her neighbor.

    A. precisely
    B. tactfully
    C. honestly
    D. positively

40. The actor's *feigned* southern accent was praised by the critics.

    A. pretended
    B. acquired
    C. unusual
    D. low-pitched

KEY (CORRECT ANSWERS)

1. B	11. D	21. A	31. C
2. A	12. A	22. A	32. B
3. D	13. C	23. C	33. A
4. A	14. A	24. B	34. D
5. C	15. B	25. D	35. C
6. D	16. D	26. D	36. B
7. C	17. A	27. C	37. A
8. A	18. D	28. D	38. D
9. B	19. C	29. A	39. B
10. C	20. B	30. A	40. A

TEST 2

DIRECTIONS: In the space provided at the right, write the letter of the word or expression that most nearly expresses the meaning of the word printed in italics.

1. *Abduct* 1.____
   - A. ruin
   - B. aid
   - C. fight
   - D. kidnap

2. *Demerit* 2.____
   - A. outcome
   - B. fault
   - C. prize
   - D. notice

3. *Mutinous* 3.____
   - A. silent
   - B. oceangoing
   - C. rebellious
   - D. miserable

4. *Negligent* 4.____
   - A. lax
   - B. desperate
   - C. cowardly
   - D. ambitious

5. *Contest* 5.____
   - A. disturb
   - B. dispute
   - C. detain
   - D. distrust

6. *Query* 6.____
   - A. wait
   - B. lose
   - C. show
   - D. ask

7. *Insidious* 7.____
   - A. treacherous
   - B. excitable
   - C. internal
   - D. distracting

8. *Palpitate* 8.____
   - A. mash
   - B. stifle
   - C. throb
   - D. pace

9. *Animosity* 9.____
   - A. hatred
   - B. interest
   - C. silliness
   - D. amusement

10. *Egotism* 10.____
    - A. sociability
    - B. aggressiveness
    - C. self-confidence
    - D. conceit

11. Bob's account of the accident *incriminated* others. 11.____
    - A. annoyed
    - B. involved
    - C. ignored
    - D. helped

177

12. When Jack left his position as chief of staff, he was completely *demoralized*.

    A. satisfied
    B. frenzied
    C. liberated
    D. disheartened

13. The architect designed a modern *edifice* of wood and red glass.

    A. framework
    B. platform
    C. structure
    D. false front

14. The speaker kept the meeting interesting with her *facetious* remarks.

    A. amusing
    B. informal
    C. personal
    D. factual

15. The new ruling set a *precedent* for all similar cases that would be tried in court.

    A. direction
    B. standard
    C. regulation
    D. test

16. The botanist wanted a picture of the tree because it was so *gnarled*.

    A. old
    B. unusual
    C. fruitful
    D. deformed

17. Harriet's *ostentatious* display of wealth is upsetting to her friends.

    A. frequent
    B. thoughtless
    C. showy
    D. unnatural

18. The answer was too *oblique* to receive full credit.

    A. indirect
    B. repetitive
    C. disorganized
    D. brief

19. The magician did the sleight-of-hand trick with remarkable *dexterity*.

    A. swiftness
    B. assurance
    C. charisma
    D. skill

20. The principal had no *qualms* about suspending the three boys for fighting.

    A. comments
    B. misgivings
    C. arguments
    D. regrets

21. *Resurrection*

    A. reassurance
    B. encouragement
    C. fascination
    D. revival

22. *Recede*

    A. take over
    B. show off
    C. hold out
    D. move back

23. *Fissure*

    A. opening
    B. path
    C. mountain
    D. landslide

24. *Delectable*

    A. carefree B. elaborate
    C. delightful D. deliberate

25. *Oblivious*

    A. understated B. unmindful
    C. untrue D. unappetizing

26. *Inevitable*

    A. unable B. forceful
    C. certain D. plain

27. *Paradox*

    A. incomplete response B. sharp comment
    C. obvious truth D. seeming contradiction

28. *Cataclysm*

    A. disaster B. deception
    C. denial D. debate

29. *Sanction*

    A. stop B. expel
    C. approve D. refund

30. *Assiduously*

    A. decidedly B. diligently
    C. randomly D. correctly

31. The judge ordered that *restitution* be provided for the robbery victims.

    A. apologies B. recognition
    C. publicity D. compensation

32. The trumpets announced the *imminent* arrival of the dignitary.

    A. approaching B. delayed
    C. unexpected D. distant

33. The shopper was *indignant* at the treatment given him by the clerk.

    A. embarrassed B. pleased
    C. angry D. surprised

34. The cook in the old diner had a *slatternly* appearance.

    A. dreary B. sloppy
    C. homey D. strange

35. The *nebulous* argument that he presented failed to explain the main issue.

    A. careful B. complex
    C. vague D. idealistic

36. The prisoner longed for the life of a *vagabond*. 36.____

   A. wanderer B. millionaire
   C. celebrity D. journalist

37. The entire neighborhood came out to see the *celestial* display. 37.____

   A. artistic B. fantastic
   C. unusual D. heavenly

38. Because the shopkeeper was upset, we were unable to *glean* the details of the robbery. 38.____

   A. connect B. gather
   C. tell D. comprehend

39. The problem rests not with her beliefs but with her excessive desire to *propagate* them. 39.____

   A. spread B. live up to
   C. protect D. justify

40. The young athlete tried to *emulate* his high school coach. 40.____

   A. obey B. assist
   C. imitate D. deceive

KEY (CORRECT ANSWERS)

1. D	11. B	21. D	31. D
2. B	12. D	22. D	32. A
3. C	13. C	23. A	33. C
4. A	14. A	24. C	34. B
5. B	15. B	25. B	35. C
6. D	16. D	26. C	36. A
7. A	17. C	27. D	37. D
8. C	18. A	28. A	38. B
9. A	19. D	29. C	39. A
10. D	20. B	30. B	40. C

TEST 3

DIRECTIONS: In the space provided at the right, write the letter of the word or expression that most nearly expresses the meaning of the word printed in italics.

1. *Intuition* 1.____
   - A. payment
   - B. faith
   - C. introduction
   - D. insight

2. *Compel* 2.____
   - A. lengthen
   - B. help
   - C. force
   - D. distract

3. *Vent* 3.____
   - A. discharge
   - B. omit
   - C. entertain
   - D. worship

4. *Cohort* 4.____
   - A. commander
   - B. companion
   - C. candidate
   - D. craftsman

5. *Ordeal* 5.____
   - A. alternate route
   - B. logical sequence
   - C. important duty
   - D. severe trial

6. *Fabrication* 6.____
   - A. addition
   - B. remedy
   - C. analysis
   - D. creation

7. *Unwitting* 7.____
   - A. ordinary
   - B. unaware
   - C. unnecessary
   - D. unadvisable

8. *Zealot* 8.____
   - A. sharp tool
   - B. worthy cause
   - C. eager person
   - D. extinct animal

9. *Indulge* 9.____
   - A. spoil
   - B. surprise
   - C. direct
   - D. compare

10. *Hamper* 10.____
    - A. offer
    - B. confuse
    - C. order
    - D. restrict

11. The first settlers in America faced a cold winter in the *vast* wilderness. 11.____
    - A. unknown
    - B. untamed
    - C. enormous
    - D. empty

181

12. Her very presence at the party *nettled* the other guests. 12._____

    A. embarrassed B. irritated
    C. puzzled   D. quieted

13. The attorney was eager to *disclose* her evidence. 13._____

    A. examine B. reorganize
    C. report   D. reveal

14. When the brakes failed, the bus nearly went off the road into a *chasm*. 14._____

    A. gorge B. field
    C. river D. wall

15. I avoid that restaurant because of its *insipid* food. 15._____

    A. spicy   B. tasteless
    C. overcooked D. expensive

16. A *malicious* person is usually unpopular. 16._____

    A. conceited B. selfish
    C. spiteful   D. stingy

17. He was able to *elude* the soldiers for only a short time. 17._____

    A. escape B. train
    C. aid   D. restrain

18. The man *denounced* his neighbor because of her political activities. 18._____

    A. avoided   B. ridiculed
    C. spied on D. condemned

19. The grapegrowers in California employ many *transient* workers. 19._____

    A. immigrant B. youthful
    C. temporary D. experienced

20. The money has been *allocated* for new school buses. 20._____

    A. set aside B. raised
    C. spent   D. borrowed

21. *Larceny* 21._____

    A. criminal   B. burning
    C. name-calling D. theft

22. *Simulate* 22._____

    A. delay   B. supply
    C. pretend D. deny

23. *Lucid* 23._____

    A. clear   B. colorful
    C. lawful D. old

24. *Remorse* 24.____
   A. anger B. regret
   C. apology D. coldness

25. *Laden* 25.____
   A. optimistic B. refined
   C. burdened D. worried

26. *Turbulence* 26.____
   A. control B. interruption
   C. renewal D. disorder

27. *Incessantly* 27.____
   A. instantly B. brilliantly
   C. respectfully D. continually

28. *Chronic* 28.____
   A. diseased B. constant
   C. aged D. unsafe

29. *Tepid* 29.____
   A. lukewarm B. eager
   C. tearful D. sharp

30. *Consensus* 30.____
   A. survey B. contract
   C. association D. agreement

31. Have you ever heard the saying, "To be *wary* is to be wise"? 31.____
   A. Thrifty B. Healthy
   C. Careful D. Industrious

32. Sherlock Holmes was noted for his superb power of *deduction*. 32.____
   A. imagination B. reasoning
   C. extrasensory perception D. concentration

33. The manager encouraged the staff to try to add to the store's *clientele*. 33.____
   A. good will B. profits
   C. customers D. variety of merchandise

34. The student was *disconcerted* when she saw her test score. 34.____
   A. upset B. assured
   C. pleased D. surprised

35. An automobile can be a *lethal* machine. 35.____
   A. expensive B. deadly
   C. essential D. magnificent

36. The general promised to *annihilate* the enemy's troops. 36.____

    A. pursue
    C. capture
    B. destroy
    D. surround

37. She is the owner of a *lucrative* construction company. 37.____

    A. small
    C. local
    B. reliable
    D. profitable

38. After Joan had completed her investigation, she realized that her *premise* was incorrect. 38.____

    A. assumption
    C. methodology
    B. conclusion
    D. information

39. During the campaign, the politicians often engaged in *acrimonious* debate. 39.____

    A. meaningless
    C. bitter
    B. brilliant
    D. loud

40. There is no value in this *sordid* film. 40.____

    A. boring
    C. experimental
    B. vile
    D. inferior

KEY (CORRECT ANSWERS)

1.	D	11.	C	21.	D	31.	C
2.	C	12.	B	22.	C	32.	B
3.	A	13.	D	23.	A	33.	C
4.	B	14.	A	24.	B	34.	A
5.	D	15.	B	25.	C	35.	B
6.	D	16.	C	26.	D	36.	B
7.	B	17.	A	27.	D	37.	D
8.	C	18.	D	28.	B	38.	A
9.	A	19.	C	29.	A	39.	C
10.	D	20.	A	30.	D	40.	B

TEST 4

DIRECTIONS: In the space provided at the right, write the letter of the word or expression that most nearly expresses the meaning of the word printed in italics.

1. *Defame*

   A. slander
   C. outwit
   B. depress
   D. arouse

   1.____

2. *Retaliation*

   A. recommendation
   C. revenge
   B. list
   D. victory

   2.____

3. *Zeal*

   A. boredom
   C. compassion
   B. enthusiasm
   D. trust

   3.____

4. *Unilateral*

   A. one-wheeled
   C. similar
   B. unanticipated
   D. one-sided

   4.____

5. *Gratuity*

   A. tip for service
   C. medal for achievement
   B. tool for printing
   D. thank you note

   5.____

6. *Bewitch*

   A. repel
   C. satisfy
   B. fascinate
   D. fear

   6.____

7. *Desist*

   A. cause
   C. help
   B. change
   D. stop

   7.____

8. *Bigotry*

   A. invention
   C. intolerance
   B. obstruction
   D. belief

   8.____

9. *Somber*

   A. gloomy
   C. lively
   B. gentle
   D. careful

   9.____

10. *Redemption*

    A. power
    C. religion
    B. sale
    D. deliverance

    10.____

11. The *eccentric* old lady loved her cats, her hats, and her tumble-down house.

    A. moody
    C. strange
    B. lovable
    D. friendly

    11.____

185

12. The author was totally displeased with the *abridged* version of his novel.

    A. televised
    B. shortened
    C. translated
    D. censored

13. He made the statement *assertively*.

    A. reluctantly
    B. hastily
    C. positively
    D. honestly

14. Because of his *inertia*, he seldom achieves his goal.

    A. temper
    B. laziness
    C. stupidity
    D. carelessness

15. The executive believes that people must be *ruthless* in order to succeed in business.

    A. powerful
    B. dishonest
    C. reckless
    D. merciless

16. The actress was described as having *mediocre* talent.

    A. ordinary
    B. uncommon
    C. excellent
    D. inferior

17. The *gaudy* dress is trimmed with pearls.

    A. elegant
    B. worn out
    C. pretty
    D. flashy

18. The class *extolled* the virtues of their teacher.

    A. listed
    B. praised
    C. apologized for
    D. explained

19. The child was both *gregarious* and hardworking in school.

    A. comfortable
    B. prompt
    C. sociable
    D. happy

20. Many *credulous* people are influenced by television advertisements to buy certain products.

    A. believing
    B. uneducated
    C. clever
    D. logical

21. *Tantalize*

    A. encourage
    B. tease
    C. satisfy
    D. quarrel

22. *Proximity*

    A. falseness
    B. correctness
    C. favor
    D. nearness

23. *Perceptible*

    A. capable
    B. likeable
    C. observable
    D. returnable

24. *Philanthropy*
    A. love of money B. love of humanity
    C. love of stamps D. love of words

25. *Havoc*
    A. respect B. danger
    C. destruction D. complications

26. *Consolidate*
    A. unite B. sympathize
    C. void D. profit

27. *Discrepancy*
    A. reduction B. restraint
    C. looseness D. difference

28. *Advocate* (verb)
    A. recommend B. supply
    C. remove D. vote

29. *Sedate*
    A. seated B. composed
    C. bored D. informal

30. *Superficial*
    A. buried B. overhead
    C. external D. important

31. Canoeing through the rapids is a *grueling* experience.
    A. exciting B. uncomfortable
    C. rewarding D. exhausting

32. He was *cognizant* of his responsibilities.
    A. aware B. afraid
    C. weary D. relieved

33. With Joe's *tenacity*, he is bound to succeed.
    A. intelligence B. luck
    C. talent D. persistence

34. When will the sales campaign be *initiated*?
    A. Approved B. Planned
    C. Started D. Tested

35. Joan's *vitality* is envied by many people.
    A. beauty B. energy
    C. ability D. popularity

36. In view of the circumstances, Jane's comment seemed *callous*.

    A. insensitive
    B. misleading
    C. kind
    D. true

37. Reading the letter left him in a *pensive* mood.

    A. calm
    B. thoughtful
    C. happy
    D. romantic

38. He answered the question *impetuously*.

    A. foolishly
    B. hastily
    C. quietly
    D. honestly

39. His *inane* suggestion fell on deaf ears.

    A. silly
    B. detailed
    C. unusual
    D. selfish

40. After being lost in the woods, Tom was *ravenous*.

    A. extremely tired
    B. extremely thirsty
    C. extremely hungry
    D. extremely angry

KEY (CORRECT ANSWERS)

1. A	11. C	21. B	31. D
2. C	12. B	22. D	32. A
3. B	13. C	23. C	33. D
4. D	14. B	24. B	34. C
5. A	15. D	25. C	35. B
6. B	16. A	26. A	36. A
7. D	17. D	27. D	37. B
8. C	18. B	28. A	38. B
9. A	19. C	29. B	39. A
10. D	20. A	30. C	40. C

WORD MEANING
EXAMINATION SECTION
TEST 1

DIRECTIONS: *In the space provided write the number of the word or phrase that most nearly expresses the meaning of the word printed in heavy black type.*

1. **induce**

    A. deceive
    B. scare
    C. ridicule
    D. cause

    1.____

2. **encore**

    A. additional performance
    B. standing ovation
    C. dramatic ending
    D. favorable review

    2.____

3. **plausible**

    A. believable
    B. circumstantial
    C. intricate
    D. unemotional

    3.____

4. **fiasco**

    A. serious undertaking
    B. complete failure
    C. long delay
    D. important observation

    4.____

5. **enhance**

    A. influence
    B. cultivate
    C. intensify
    D. establish

    5.____

6. **arrogantly**

    A. expertly
    B. cleverly
    C. overbearingly
    D. recklessly

    6.____

7. **tainted**

    A. contaminated
    B. deflated
    C. softened
    D. adapted

    7.____

8. **delve**

    A. prepare for
    B. apply to
    C. bring up
    D. dig into

    8.____

9. **maim**

    A. mutilate
    B. misuse
    C. betray
    D. prevent

    9.____

10. **jocular**

    A. manly
    B. lucky
    C. comical
    D. slippery

    10.____

189

11. Many people with physical disabilities have learned to **transcend** their limitations.   11.____

    A. forget about   C. accept
    B. rise above   D. exploit

12. According to the review, the leading actress gave a **lackluster** performance.   12.____

    A. powerful   C. shocking
    B. sensitive   D. dull

13. She wondered if her employer would **sanction** her actions.   13.____

    A. discover   C. remember
    B. permit   D. understand

14. Do you know if she is Jane's **ally**?   14.____

    A. supervisor   C. substitute
    B. supporter   D. beneficiary

15. The woman spoke **imperiously** to the young boy.   15.____

    A. in a domineering manner
    B. persuasively
    C. politely
    D. with gentle patience

16. The executive behaved in an **omnipotent** manner.   16.____

    A. dignified   C. all-powerful
    B. optimistic   D. supportive

17. The lawyer's questions **unnerved** the witness.   17.____

    A. upset   C. challenged
    B. misled   D. embarrassed

18. She was **scrupulous** in the care of her garden.   18.____

    A. imaginative   C. inconsistent
    B. precise   D. unsurpassed

19. His job was to **expedite** the manufacturing process.   19.____

    A. check on   C. oversee
    B. design   D. speed up

20. The announcement was delivered in a **guttural** voice.   20.____

    A. clear   C. authoritative
    B. loud   D. harsh

KEY (CORRECT ANSWERS)

1.	D	11.	B
2.	A	12.	D
3.	A	13.	B
4.	B	14.	B
5.	C	15.	A
6.	C	16.	C
7.	A	17.	A
8.	D	18.	B
9.	A	19.	D
10.	C	20.	D

TEST 2

DIRECTIONS: In the space provided write the number of the word or phrase that most nearly expresses the meaning of the word printed in heavy black type.

1. **laxity**   1.____
   - A. carelessness
   - B. bitterness
   - C. sarcasm
   - D. conviction

2. **nurture**   2.____
   - A. rescue
   - B. arrange
   - C. plow
   - D. foster

3. **barrage**   3.____
   - A. betrayal
   - B. attack
   - C. expression
   - D. absence

4. **optimum**   4.____
   - A. dynamic
   - B. enjoyable
   - C. most favorable
   - D. very sincere

5. **hinder**   5.____
   - A. disperse
   - B. quit
   - C. throw away
   - D. interfere with

6. **surcease**   6.____
   - A. end
   - B. trouble
   - C. laughter
   - D. doubt

7. **sporadically**   7.____
   - A. previously
   - B. occasionally
   - C. chronologically
   - D. presently

8. **feasible**   8.____
   - A. mechanical
   - B. hesitant
   - C. likely
   - D. tolerant

9. **wily**   9.____
   - A. quick
   - B. crafty
   - C. skilled
   - D. shy

10. **defunct**   10.____
    - A. extinct
    - B. balanced
    - C. saddened
    - D. degraded

11. She **brazenly** presented her opinion to the group.

    A. nervously
    B. cautiously
    C. honestly
    D. boldly

12. Several **irate** parents attended the school board meeting.

    A. influential
    B. angry
    C. distressed
    D. noisy

13. The prisoner was judged to be **incorrigible.**

    A. incapable of being reformed
    B. unlikely to cause trouble
    C. unable to understand the charges
    D. ineligible for parole

14. Most people are happy with their **niche** in life.

    A. goals
    B. position
    C. recognition
    D. accomplishments

15. The attorney stood up to **illuminate** the points of the argument.

    A. list
    B. repeat
    C. clarify
    D. deny

16. The swimmer **flailed** away in the swift current.

    A. plunged forward
    B. thrashed about
    C. shouted for help
    D. gasped for air

17. He was noted for his **philanthropic** interests.

    A. religious
    B. athletic
    C. intellectual
    D. humanitarian

18. In some cultures, kings were **deified.**

    A. selected for life
    B. believed to be infallible
    C. buried with their possessions
    D. worshiped as gods

19. The criminal's **guise** surprised the police.

    A. skill
    B. intelligence
    C. appearance
    D. attitude

20. The climbers knew they could **traverse** the glacier.

    A. go across
    B. encounter
    C. explore
    D. tunnel through

KEY (CORRECT ANSWERS)

1. A
2. D
3. B
4. C
5. D

6. A
7. B
8. C
9. B
10. A

11. D
12. B
13. A
14. B
15. C

16. B
17. D
18. D
19. C
20. A

TEST 3

DIRECTIONS: *In the space provided write the number of the word or phrase that most nearly expresses the meaning of the word printed in heavy black type.*

1. **rouse**   1.____
    - A. rescue
    - B. misinform
    - C. awaken
    - D. eliminate

2. **ravenously**   2.____
    - A. hungrily
    - B. fearfully
    - C. carelessly
    - D. angrily

3. **decrepit**   3.____
    - A. poor
    - B. humble
    - C. complaining
    - D. weak

4. **quandary**   4.____
    - A. dilemma
    - B. journey
    - C. accident
    - D. contest

5. **trauma**   5.____
    - A. crime
    - B. injury
    - C. failure
    - D. invasion

6. **fortitude**   6.____
    - A. strength of mind
    - B. generosity of spirit
    - C. grace of movement
    - D. ease of understanding

7. **stark**   7.____
    - A. remote
    - B. closed
    - C. barren
    - D. foreign

8. **pinnacle**   8.____
    - A. convenient shelter
    - B. wooded area
    - C. secluded beach
    - D. lofty peak

9. **allot**   9.____
    - A. scheme
    - B. distribute
    - C. review
    - D. multiply

10. **convivial**   10.____
    - A. sociable
    - B. important
    - C. wealthy
    - D. lucky

11. As a result of illness, he lost his **equilibrium**. 11.____

    A. balance C. strength
    B. memory D. vitality

12. The publicity about the politician was **demeaning**. 12.____

    A. unreliable C. incriminating
    B. degrading D. contradictory

13. The resort was known for its **ambience**. 13.____

    A. convenient location B. recreational facilities
    C. healthful climate D. distinct atmosphere

14. The student felt like a **nonentity** in the new school. 14.____

    A. an inexperienced person B. an insignificant person
    C. an incompetent person D. an unpopular person

15. When the scientist switched on the machine, it began to **oscillate**. 15.____

    A. hum C. vibrate
    B. glow D. spark

16. In ancient times, people **invoked** their gods in elaborate ceremonies. 16.____

    A. called upon C. thanked
    B. sacrificed to D. pacified

17. At the **commencement** of the festivities, the mayor spoke to the crowd. 17.____

    A. close C. climax
    B. midpoint D. beginning

18. The student had a reputation for telling **blatant** lies. 18.____

    A. harmless C. imaginative
    B. obvious D. elaborate

19. The child's **astute** answer surprised his father. 19.____

    A. rude C. humorous
    B. unfeeling D. shrewd

20. The tiger lay **languorously** in the shadow of a large boulder. 20.____

    A. sluggishly C. expectantly
    B. patiently D. silently

KEY (CORRECT ANSWERS)

1.	C	11.	A
2.	A	12.	B
3.	D	13.	D
4.	A	14.	B
5.	B	15.	C
6.	A	16.	A
7.	C	17.	D
8.	D	18.	B
9.	B	19.	D
10.	A	20.	A

TEST 4

DIRECTIONS: *In the space provided write the number of the word or phrase that most nearly expresses the meaning of the word printed in heavy black type.*

1. **detest**
   - A. deny
   - B. specify
   - C. examine
   - D. loathe

2. **fracas**
   - A. feast
   - B. brawl
   - C. search
   - D. fracture

3. **juncture**
   - A. decision
   - B. climax
   - C. connection
   - D. emergency

4. **constrict**
   - A. make smooth
   - B. make narrow
   - C. make flexible
   - D. make flat

5. **meticulous**
   - A. careful of details
   - B. considerate of others
   - C. worthy of honor
   - D. taken for granted

6. **absolve**
   - A. engage
   - B. relate
   - C. suggest
   - D. pardon

7. **wrath**
   - A. intense fear
   - B. deep despair
   - C. bitter resentment
   - D. fierce anger

8. **zenith**
   - A. summit
   - B. path
   - C. flight
   - D. goal

9. **clandestine**
   - A. secret
   - B. silent
   - C. strange
   - D. sacred

10. **genial**
    - A. desirable
    - B. generous
    - C. friendly
    - D. happy

11. He was **grievously** ill.

    A. seriously
    B. frequently
    C. constantly
    D. fatally

    11._____

12. She was able to devise a **viable** solution to the plan.

    A. unique
    B. workable
    C. novel
    D. simple

    12._____

13. The newspaper reported the Senate's **nullification** of the treaty.

    A. postponement
    B. revision
    C. invalidation
    D. confirmation

    13._____

14. One reason gold is used for jewelry is that it is very **malleable**.

    A. delicate
    B. shiny
    C. beautiful
    D. pliable

    14._____

15. The President listened to the news with **equanimity**.

    A. disbelief
    B. composure
    C. amazement
    D. annoyance

    15._____

16. The child **recoiled** when the lightning flashed.

    A. trembled
    B. fled
    C. flinched
    D. cried

    16._____

17. The scientist hoped to **eradicate** the bacteria that caused the disease.

    A. destroy
    B. identify
    C. study
    D. alter

    17._____

18. The offender received a hearing that was **impartial**.

    A. speedy
    B. private
    C. preliminary
    D. fair

    18._____

19. The judge directed the jury to ignore the witness' **scathing** remarks.

    A. obviously rehearsed
    B. totally irrelevant
    C. bitterly severe
    D. highly opinionated

    19._____

20. The **russet** leaves were piled by the roadway.

    A. newly fallen
    B. wet
    C. decaying
    D. reddish-brown

    20._____

KEY (CORRECT ANSWERS)

1.	D	11.	A
2.	B	12.	B
3.	C	13.	C
4.	B	14.	D
5.	A	15.	B
6.	D	16.	C
7.	D	17.	A
8.	A	18.	D
9.	A	19.	C
10.	C	20.	D

TEST 5

DIRECTIONS: *In the space provided write the number of the word or phrase that most nearly expresses the meaning of the word printed in heavy black type.*

1. **variance**

    A. authority
    B. nuisance
    C. regulation
    D. difference

    1.____

2. **entail**

    A. produce
    B. involve
    C. emphasize
    D. forbid

    2.____

3. **trudge**

    A. retreat
    B. slouch
    C. plod
    D. scurry

    3.____

4. **acme**

    A. highest point
    B. final proposal
    C. detailed explanation
    D. preliminary investigation

    4.____

5. **vanquish**

    A. clean
    B. criticize
    C. comfort
    D. conquer

    5.____

6. **salve**

    A. gauge
    B. ointment
    C. scar
    D. bandage

    6.____

7. **repress**

    A. insult
    B. disturb
    C. subdue
    D. refuse

    7.____

8. **trifling**

    A. useless
    B. insignificant
    C. grotesque
    D. dull

    8.____

9. **profoundly**

    A. deeply
    B. anxiously
    C. pleasantly
    D. loudly

    9.____

10. **insatiable**

    A. envious
    B. coarse
    C. disgusting
    D. greedy

    10.____

11. The young man had a **debonair** attitude toward life.

    A. lighthearted C. childlike
    B. pessimistic D. cautious

12. After so many years of war, the people held little hope for any **armistice**.

    A. victory C. independence
    B. election D. truce

13. The judge decided to **mitigate** the criminal's sentence.

    A. review C. lessen
    B. overrule D. postpone

14. The teacher asked the **recalcitrant** students to sit down.

    A. tardy C. unhappy
    B. unruly D. eager

15. The teacher presented a **synopsis** of the play to the class.

    A. critique C. summary
    B. history D. segment

16. **Dissidence** is not usually tolerated by dictators.

    A. disagreement C. desertion
    B. disorganization D. democracy

17. No one could **mollify** the lost child.

    A. identify C. approach
    B. understand D. soothe

18. The writing was poetic as well as **utilitarian**.

    A. creative C. witty
    B. entertaining D. useful

19. She was **inundated** by the work that had been assigned to her.

    A. overwhelmed C. astounded
    B. discouraged D. inspired

20. The exconvicts were engaged in a number of **nefarious** actions.

    A. pessimistic C. wicked
    B. wholesome D. regrettable

KEY (CORRECT ANSWERS)

1. D
2. B
3. C
4. A
5. D

6. B
7. C
8. B
9. A
10. D

11. A
12. D
13. C
14. B
15. C

16. A
17. D
18. D
19. A
20. C

TEST 6

DIRECTIONS: In the space provided write the number of the word or phrase that most nearly expresses the meaning of the word printed in heavy black type.

1. **desolate**
   - A. pitiful
   - B. displeased
   - C. sensitive
   - D. lonely

2. **poise**
   - A. maturity
   - B. self-assurance
   - C. good humor
   - D. intelligence

3. **reparation**
   - A. statement of fact
   - B. payment for damage
   - C. expression of sorrow
   - D. regulation of trade

4. **indisputably**
   - A. unfairly
   - B. unclearly
   - C. illogically
   - D. undeniably

5. **atrocious**
   - A. horrifying
   - B. forceful
   - C. furious
   - D. ridiculous

6. **misconstrue**
   - A. misinform
   - B. misplace
   - C. misunderstand
   - D. mishandle

7. **wield**
   - A. argue loudly
   - B. handle skillfully
   - C. change needlessly
   - D. test periodically

8. **rue**
   - A. relive
   - B. regain
   - C. recall
   - D. regret

9. **ashen**
   - A. pale
   - B. cowardly
   - C. deformed
   - D. bitter

10. **piety**
    - A. class
    - B. devoutness
    - C. affection
    - D. control

11. The missionary received an award for her **benevolent** work.

    A. religious
    B. original
    C. charitable
    D. scholarly

12. The waiter was pleased by the **gratuity** he had received.

    A. raise
    B. promotion
    C. advice
    D. tip

13. The candidate's latest **escapade** was reported in the newspaper.

    A. inspiring speech
    B. political blunder
    C. reckless adventure
    D. unexpected achievement

14.]The committee decided that the entire program had to be **revamped**.

    A. revised
    B. discarded
    C. studied
    D. rescheduled

15. The police officer quickly **assayed** the situation at hand.

    A. reported
    B. recognized
    C. analyzed
    D. observed

16. The audience began to **badger** the speaker.

    A. heckle
    B. ignore
    C. applaud
    D. interrupt

17. Her **avarice** was so great that it ruled her life.

    A. despair
    B. greed
    C. fear
    D. bitterness

18. Much of the information he provided was **superfluous**.

    A. illogical
    B. inaccurate
    C. biased
    D. nonessential

19. Reformed smokers sometimes become **fanatic** about the habits of people who continue to smoke.

    A. critical
    B. overly sympathetic
    C. unreasonably insistent
    D. disinterested

20. He was instrumental in forming the new **coalition**.

    A. theory
    B. temporary alliance
    C. international organization
    D. schedule

KEY (CORRECT ANSWERS)

1. D
2. B
3. B
4. D
5. A

6. C
7. B
8. D
9. A
10. B

11. C
12. D
13. C
14. A
15. C

16. A
17. B
18. D
19. C
20. B

TEST 7

DIRECTIONS: In the space provided write the number of the word or phrase that most nearly expresses the meaning of the word printed in heavy black type.

1. **fallible**
   - A. able to move quickly
   - B. well educated
   - C. capable of error
   - D. easily angered

2. **aspire**
   - A. construct
   - B. revise
   - C. ask about
   - D. yearn for

3. **virtually**
   - A. apparently
   - B. completely
   - C. nearly
   - D. repetitiously

4. **melancholy**
   - A. thoughtful
   - B. hopeful
   - C. sad
   - D. angry

5. **beguile**
   - A. annoy
   - B. condemn
   - C. deceive
   - D. encourage

6. **lament**
   - A. grieve
   - B. infiltrate
   - C. disable
   - D. labor

7. **appease**
   - A. argue
   - B. pacify
   - C. refuse
   - D. entertain

8. **amnesty**
   - A. pardon
   - B. treason
   - C. fatigue
   - D. comfort

9. **unscrupulous**
   - A. immoderate
   - B. intolerant
   - C. unemotional
   - D. unprincipled

10. **genuine**
    - A. refined
    - B. antiquated
    - C. sincere
    - D. reserved

11. The customer was annoyed by the salesclerk's **impertinent** remark.

    A. insensitive
    B. cross
    C. silly
    D. rude

12. She was not aware of the **ramification** of her proposal.

    A. cost
    B. scope
    C. consequence
    D. inappropriateness

13. The prince decided to **abdicate** his claim to the throne.

    A. defend
    B. give up
    C. clarify
    D. strengthen

14. He revealed his **craven** nature in times of danger.

    A. cowardly
    B. hypocritical
    C. devious
    D. savage

15. The speaker's message seemed unnecessarily **morose**.

    A. disrespectful
    B. scolding
    C. bitter
    D. gloomy

16. The **altercation** took place on the bus.

    A. long delay
    B. noisy quarrel
    C. serious accident
    D. first meeting

17. Her **unassuming** manner hid a will of iron.

    A. patient
    B. charming
    C. modest
    D. graceful

18. His statements were so **illusive** that they did not help me in any way.

    A. unworkable
    B. ridiculous
    C. deceptive
    D. brief

19. Art critics labeled the sculpture **farcical**.

    A. inventive
    B. absurd
    C. fashionable
    D. simplistic

20. The **entreaty** was ignored by the judge.

    A. plea
    B. agreement
    C. remark
    D. decision

KEY (CORRECT ANSWERS)

1. C
2. D
3. C
4. C
5. C

6. A
7. B
8. A
9. D
10. C

11. D
12. C
13. B
14. A
15. D

16. B
17. C
18. C
19. B
20. A

TEST 8

DIRECTIONS: *In the space provided write the number of the word or phrase that most nearly expresses the meaning of the word printed in heavy black type.*

1. **diffuse**
    - A. censor
    - B. focus
    - C. ignore
    - D. scatter

2. **skulk**
    - A. dash
    - B. lurk
    - C. rest
    - D. begin

3. **consecrate**
    - A. sanctify
    - B. provide
    - C. enlist
    - D. follow

4. **ignoble**
    - A. dishonorable
    - B. unknowing
    - C. foreboding
    - D. suspicious

5. **cache**
    - A. meeting room
    - B. hiding place
    - C. inscription
    - D. compromise

6. **bleary**
    - A. dark
    - B. rough
    - C. blurred
    - D. silvery

7. **facet**
    - A. error
    - B. curiosity
    - C. aspect
    - D. event

8. **loquacious**
    - A. temperamental
    - B. insistent
    - C. talkative
    - D. nervous

9. **averse**
    - A. enthusiastic
    - B. careful
    - C. unsure
    - D. opposed

10. **azure**
    - A. blue
    - B. gray
    - C. pink
    - D. violet

11. After a while, the blood from his wound began to **congeal.**
    - A. flow
    - B. smell
    - C. darken
    - D. thicken

12. The player's comments **incensed** the football coach. 12.____

    A. confused
    B. angered
    C. interrupted
    D. threatened

13. Winning an election often depends upon handling the campaign with **finesse**. 13.____

    A. skill
    B. efficiency
    C. humor
    D. intelligence

14. The **adjunct** professor helped with the overload of classes. 14.____

    A. orderly
    B. expert
    C. additional
    D. experienced

15. We were amused by her **madcap** behavior. 15.____

    A. childish
    B. impulsive
    C. flirtatious
    D. studious

16. Her facial expression **belied** the meaning of her words. 16.____

    A. misrepresented
    B. conveyed
    C. diminished
    D. accentuated

17. Many people in the world are living in **squalor**. 17.____

    A. anger and hatred
    B. danger and fear
    C. poverty and filth
    D. disfavor and bondage

18. I cannot work with that **incessant** noise in the background. 18.____

    A. unbearable
    B. irritating
    C. loud
    D. continuous

19. Celebrities are often asked to **endorse** products shown on television. 19.____

    A. sell
    B. demonstrate
    C. approve
    D. describe

20. The speaker used several **anecdotes** during his presentation. 20.____

    A. stories
    B. related works
    C. slides
    D. unrelated comments

KEY (CORRECT ANSWERS)

1. D
2. B
3. A
4. A
5. B

6. C
7. C
8. C
9. D
10. A

11. D
12. B
13. A
14. C
15. B

16. A
17. C
18. D
19. C
20. A

TEST 9

DIRECTIONS: In the space provided write the number of the word or phrase that most nearly expresses the meaning of the word printed in heavy black type.

1. **incognito**
   - A. famous
   - B. temporary
   - C. impossible
   - D. disguised

   1.____

2. **dynamically**
   - A. persistently
   - B. energetically
   - C. excitedly
   - D. bravely

   2.____

3. **rectify**
   - A. reverse
   - B. evaluate
   - C. correct
   - D. defend

   3.____

4. **grapple**
   - A. seize
   - B. understand
   - C. acknowledge
   - D. impress

   4.____

5. **crestfallen**
   - A. dejected
   - B. insincere
   - C. disrespectful
   - D. untidy

   5.____

6. **writhe**
   - A. deprive
   - B. twist
   - C. annoy
   - D. attach

   6.____

7. **garish**
   - A. inferior
   - B. irregular
   - C. destructive
   - D. gaudy

   7.____

8. **nepotism**
   - A. patriotism
   - B. favoritism
   - C. heroism
   - D. barbarism

   8.____

9. **heretical**
   - A. attempting to deceive
   - C. lacking knowledge of the facts
   - B. inclined to be argumentative
   - D. contrary to accepted belief

   9.____

10. **subtleties**
    - A. fine points
    - B. main ideas
    - C. inconsistencies
    - D. inaccuracies

    10.____

11. The lawyer's **prestige** earned her a nomination as a judge.

    A. experience
    B. knowledge
    C. prominence
    D. training

12. The family was **euphoric** after winning the lottery.

    A. joyful
    B. wealthy
    C. famous
    D. thankful

13. Working after school **precludes** my participation in sports.

    A. precedes
    B. prevents
    C. reduces
    D. supports

14. The meaning of that statement is **ambiguous**.

    A. incomplete
    B. unimportant
    C. lost
    D. vague

15. The children copied the passages **verbatim**.

    A. without understanding them
    B. in careful handwriting
    C. from dictation
    D. word for word

16. Some states have a **reciprocal** agreement for issuing drivers' licenses.

    A. compromise
    B. legal
    C. mutual
    D. controversial

17. The decision about the proposed legislation was **deferred**.

    A. altered
    B. approved
    C. defended
    D. delayed

18. The guide warned us about the dangerous **precipice**.

    A. cliff
    B. trail
    C. cave
    D. ravine

19. The elderly woman was amazed by the **audacity** of the child.

    A. courtesy
    B. boldness
    C. obedience
    D. wisdom

20. The teacher reluctantly **acquiesced** to the students' request for less homework.

    A. replied
    B. objected
    C. listened
    D. consented

KEY (CORRECT ANSWERS)

1.	D	11.	C
2.	B	12.	A
3.	C	13.	B
4.	A	14.	D
5.	A	15.	D
6.	B	16.	C
7.	D	17.	D
8.	B	18.	A
9.	D	19.	B
10.	A	20.	D

TEST 10

DIRECTIONS: *In the space provided write the number of the word or phrase that most nearly expresses the meaning of the word printed in heavy black type.*

1. **preferential**
    - A. daily
    - B. limited
    - C. constant
    - D. special

2. **abortive**
    - A. mature
    - B. preoccupied
    - C. unsuccessful
    - D. unreliable

3. **idiosyncrasy**
    - A. personal peculiarity
    - B. professional integrity
    - C. traditional morality
    - D. supernatural ability

4. **doldrums**
    - A. unreasonable fears
    - B. low spirits
    - C. rare diseases
    - D. unhappy memories

5. **lethargic**
    - A. empty
    - B. worried
    - C. unprepared
    - D. sluggish

6. **occult**
    - A. frightening
    - B. complex
    - C. mysterious
    - D. distant

7. **coagulate**
    - A. strangle
    - B. deny
    - C. greet
    - D. clot

8. **insubordination**
    - A. disobedience
    - B. humiliation
    - C. carelessness
    - D. rejection

9. **dissent**
    - A. discourage
    - B. discount
    - C. disagree
    - D. discard

10. **allude**
    - A. contain
    - B. refer
    - C. allow
    - D. compose

11. The arguments presented against smoking are **incontrovertible**.

    A. beyond dispute
    B. in need of correction
    C. beyond comprehension
    D. unable to be proved

12. Her conclusions were **indubitably** original.

    A. unusually
    B. unquestionably
    C. brilliantly
    D. authentically

13. The lawyer urged his client to **amend** the statement he had planned to make.

    A. prove
    B. change
    C. reconsider
    D. withdraw

14. The seven-year-old violinist was **precocious** for her age.

    A. extremely self-disciplined
    B. highly sensitive
    C. unusually advanced
    D. very well trained

15. The water in the wooden bucket began to **stagnate** after a few days.

    A. become foul
    B. leak out
    C. evaporate
    D. soak in

16. The judge attempted to **conciliate** the parties in the dispute.

    A. punish
    B. separate
    C. persuade
    D. pacify

17. After many hours of negotiation, the two sides had reached an **impasse**.

    A. identification of issues
    B. explanation of both viewpoints
    C. argument over the next step
    D. inability to agree

18. The acrobat's **lithe** movements amazed the crowd.

    A. complicated
    B. rapid
    C. flexible
    D. dreamlike

19. The contest rules did not allow **facsimiles** to be submitted.

    A. exact copies
    B. factual statements
    C. late entries
    D. incomplete forms

20. His **demeanor** left much to be desired.

    A. clothing
    B. manner
    C. judgment
    D. taste

KEY (CORRECT ANSWERS)

1.	D	11.	A
2.	C	12.	B
3.	A	13.	B
4.	B	14.	C
5.	D	15.	A
6.	C	16.	D
7.	D	17.	D
8.	A	18.	C
9.	C	19.	A
10.	B	20.	B

ANTONYMS/OPPOSITES
EXAMINATION SECTION
TEST 1

DIRECTIONS: Each question below consists of a word printed in capital letters, followed by five words or phrases lettered A through E. Choose the lettered word or phrase that is *most nearly* OPPOSITE in meaning to the word in capital letters. *PRINT THE LETTER OF THE CORRECT ANSWER IN THE SPACE AT THE RIGHT.*

1. ACRID
   - A. smoky
   - B. withered
   - C. sharp
   - D. mild
   - E. acerb

2. ALLERGY
   - A. extreme sensitivity
   - B. distaste
   - C. sleepiness
   - D. suppressed desire
   - E. unsusceptibility

3. AMBIGUOUS
   - A. acoustic
   - B. ambivalent
   - C. equivocal
   - D. imitating
   - E. succinct

4. AMELIORATE
   - A. bring together
   - B. settle a dispute
   - C. worsen
   - D. improve
   - E. amend

5. AUGMENT
   - A. sever
   - B. disperse
   - C. increase
   - D. diminish
   - E. argue

6. BANAL
   - A. sarcastic
   - B. trite
   - C. novel
   - D. futuristic
   - E. sagacious

7. BEATIFY
   - A. make lovely
   - B. desecrate
   - C. make happy
   - D. restore
   - E. hallow

8. BOURGEOIS
   - A. middle-class citizen
   - B. capital letters
   - C. swollen streams
   - D. nobility
   - E. peasant

9. BROMIDE
   - A. vegetable
   - B. petty bribe
   - C. pamphlet
   - D. skin abrasion
   - E. epigram

10. BRING

    A. fetch B. transfer C. relate
    D. suggest E. dispatch

11. CAPRICIOUS

    A. fickle B. fault-finding C. sneering
    D. dominating E. resolve

12. CASUAL

    A. watery B. fated C. fortuitous
    D. aromatic E. moving

13. CHOLERIC

    A. dignified B. high-tempered C. gloomy
    D. unexcitable E. caustic

14. CIRCULAR

    A. muscular B. oblique C. grouped
    D. pivotal E. incongruous

15. CIRCUMVENT

    A. succor B. reserve C. fortify
    D. surround E. delude

16. COMPASSIONATE

    A. pitiful B. merciful C. ruthless
    D. reluctant E. pietistic

17. COMPLIANCE

    A. violation B. regulation C. attendance
    D. submission E. conformance

18. CONDIGN

    A. punishable B. scheming C. undeserved
    D. merited E. condemn

19. CONDONE

    A. demand payment B. express sympathy C. forget
    D. revenge E. forgive

20. COPE

    A. fail in striving B. contend on equal terms
    C. plug with soft material D. crown with laurel
    E. compare with others

21. DECOROUS

    A. unseemly B. proper C. low cut
    D. in groups of ten E. deteriorating

22. DESPONDENT

    A. powdery   B. bent   C. optional
    D. artificial   E. elated

22._____

23. DESULTORY

    A. pompous   B. methodical   C. rambling
    D. oppressively hot   E. cursory

23._____

24. DETONATE

    A. explode   B. deafen   C. muffle
    D. fizzle out   E. destroy

24._____

25. DISCIPLE

    A. impostor   B. follower   C. antagonist
    D. paragon   E. colleague

25._____

KEYS (CORRECT ANSWERS)

1.	D	11.	E
2.	E	12.	B
3.	E	13.	D
4.	C	14.	B
5.	D	15.	A
6.	C	16.	C
7.	B	17.	A
8.	E	18.	C
9.	E	19.	D
10.	E	20.	A

21. A
22. E
23. B
24. C
25. C

TEST 2

DIRECTIONS: Each question below consists of a word printed in capital letters, followed by five words or phrases lettered A through E. Choose the lettered word or phrase that is *most nearly* OPPOSITE in meaning to the word in capital letters. *PRINT THE LETTER OF THE CORRECT ANSWER IN THE SPACE AT THE RIGHT.*

1. DISCREET
   - A. cautious
   - B. chary
   - C. prudent
   - D. distinct
   - E. temerarious

2. DISINTER
   - A. dig up from a grave
   - B. lack interest
   - C. interrupt
   - D. inject between muscles
   - E. entomb

3. DOGGEREL
   - A. trivial verse
   - B. small canine species
   - C. stubborn behavior
   - D. sophisticated poetry
   - E. manger

4. DOLE OUT
   - A. squander
   - B. distribute piecemeal
   - C. control
   - D. deny alms
   - E. hoard

5. DOMINEERING
   - A. dictatorial
   - B. pliant
   - C. considerate
   - D. unsympathetic
   - E. recreant

6. ELEGY
   - A. inheritance
   - B. burnt offering
   - C. violin obbligato
   - D. dirge
   - E. paean

7. ELICIT
   - A. concoct with alcohol
   - B. draw out
   - C. compel approval
   - D. request sharply
   - E. ignite

8. EMOLLIENT
   - A. salve
   - B. monument
   - C. tariff charge
   - D. extra tip
   - E. abrasive

9. ENCORE
   - A. intermission
   - B. termination
   - C. heart of the matter
   - D. repetition
   - E. variation

10. ENERVATE
    - A. stumble
    - B. devitalize
    - C. stimulate
    - D. rejoice
    - E. impede

11. EXPIATION   11._____
    A. reprobation   B. clarification   C. failure
    D. atonement   E. interpretation

12. FABULOUS   12._____
    A. wealthy   B. impressionistic   C. realistic
    D. legendary   E. fictional

13. FAIRWAY   13._____
    A. airplane landing field   B. golf greensward   C. captain's private quarters
    D. entrance to ferry slip   E. coppice

14. FEASIBLE   14._____
    A. garish   B. festive   C. theoretical
    D. practicable   E. pertinent

15. FIERY   15._____
    A. vehement   B. irritable   C. restive
    D. gay   E. indifferent

16. FLORID   16._____
    A. flowing   B. livid   C. blotchy
    D. ruddy   E. over-heated

17. FLOUT   17._____
    A. move   B. mock   C. obey
    D. defy   E. flog

18. FOREGO   18._____
    A. prosecute   B. align   C. renounce
    D. look forward   E. over-heated

19. FURTIVE   19._____
    A. fleeing   B. hairy   C. glancing
    D. stealthy   E. ingenuous

20. GARBLE   20._____
    A. substantiate   B. garnish   C. mutilate
    D. unravel   E. embroider

21. GARRULOUS   21._____
    A. talkative   B. quarrelsome   C. snarling
    D. laconic   E. ungainly

22. GOSSAMER   22._____
    A. sleezy   B. dusty   C. gauzy
    D. unbreakable   E. zephyr-like

23. GOURMAND

   A. greedy eater
   B. epicure
   C. hungry person
   D. ascetic
   E. fried pumpkin shell

24. GRIEVOUS

   A. rutty
   B. gratifying
   C. sorrowful
   D. vicious
   E. unmentionable

25. GRIMACE

   A. happy smile
   B. fruit sherbet
   C. twisting of the countenance
   D. fine quality silk
   E. sneer

KEYS (CORRECT ANSWERS)

1. E
2. E
3. D
4. A
5. B

6. E
7. D
8. E
9. B
10. C

11. A
12. C
13. E
14. C
15. E

16. B
17. C
18. A
19. E
20. A

21. D
22. D
23. D
24. B
25. A

TEST 3

DIRECTIONS: Each question below consists of a word printed in capital letters, followed by five words or phrases lettered A through E. Choose the lettered word or phrase that is *most nearly* OPPOSITE in meaning to the word in capital letters. *PRINT THE LETTER OF THE CORRECT ANSWER IN THE SPACE AT THE RIGHT.*

1. HEINOUS
   - A. criminal
   - B. elevated
   - C. inhuman
   - D. flagrant
   - E. moderate

   1.____

2. HUE
   - A. tint
   - B. shade
   - C. tone
   - D. tinge
   - E. etiolation

   2.____

3. IMMUNITY
   - A. protection against accident
   - B. exemption
   - C. freedom from disease
   - D. dispensation
   - E. tendency

   3.____

4. IMPLICIT
   - A. directly stated
   - B. understood though not expressed
   - C. omitted entirely by chance
   - D. stated but not for publication
   - E. inherent

   4.____

5. IMPUTE
   - A. insult
   - B. contradict
   - C. ascribe
   - D. question
   - E. refer

   5.____

6. INCIPIENT
   - A. tasteless
   - B. criminal
   - C. beginning
   - D. diseased
   - E. terminal

   6.____

7. INGENUOUS
   - A. guileful
   - B. naive
   - C. frank
   - D. uncertain
   - E. jealous

   7.____

8. INIQUITOUS
   - A. awesome
   - B. unequal
   - C. wicked
   - D. present everywhere
   - E. exemplary

   8.____

9. INTERMITTENT
   - A. continuing without break
   - B. occurring at intervals
   - C. persistently noisy
   - D. gradually subdued
   - E. intermediate

   9.____

10. INTRANSIGENT
    A. utterly fearless   B. irreconcilable   C. invalid
    D. not transferable   E. tractable

11. INTREPID
    A. fearful   B. uneasy   C. dauntless
    D. stumbling   E. insistent

12. INURE
    A. maim   B. entice   C. deplete
    D. toughen   E. endure

13. INVOKE
    A. provoke   B. denounce   C. slanderous
    D. address in prayer   E. evoke

14. NOSTALGIA
    A. homesickness   B. inertia   C. gloominess
    D. nasal catarrh   E. wanderlust

15. OCCULT
    A. abstract   B. manifest   C. secret
    D. oriental   E. acute

16. ONEROUS
    A. unwanted   B. impossible   C. delicate
    D. burdensome   E. facile

17. OPULENT
    A. expensive   B. oily   C. crafty
    D. profuse   E. jejune

18. ORDINANCE
    A. excess weight   B. anarchy   C. law
    D. military supplies   E. mound of filth

19. ORTHOGRAPHY
    A. correct accent   B. choice of words   C. misspelling
    D. derivation of words   E. clear enunciation

20. PAROCHIAL
    A. limited in range   B. sacred   C. stubborn
    D. objective   E. easily manageable

21. PEREMPTORY
    A. trifling   B. compliant   C. arbitrary
    D. binding   E. camouflaged

22. PERVADE

    A. pass along
    C. convince at length
    E. confine
    B. escape quietly
    D. to be diffused throughout

23. PERVERSITY

    A. cruelty
    D. adherent
    B. miserliness
    E. frugality
    C. conformity

24. PHLEGMATIC

    A. stolid
    D. sentient
    B. figurative
    E. substantial
    C. aphasic

25. POIGNANT

    A. melancholy
    D. keen
    B. soothing
    E. reluctant
    C. doubtful

KEYS (CORRECT ANSWERS)

1. B	11. A
2. E	12. C
3. E	13. B
4. A	14. E
5. B	15. B
6. E	16. E
7. A	17. E
8. E	18. B
9. A	19. C
10. E	20. D

21. B
22. E
23. C
24. D
25. B

TEST 4

DIRECTIONS: Each question below consists of a word printed in capital letters, followed by five words or phrases lettered A through E. Choose the lettered word or phrase that is *most nearly* OPPOSITE in meaning to the word in capital letters. *PRINT THE LETTER OF THE CORRECT ANSWER IN THE SPACE AT THE RIGHT.*

1. PRODIGIOUS
   - A. extraordinary
   - B. commonplace
   - C. profound
   - D. prehistoric
   - E. infinitesmal

   1.____

2. PUERILE
   - A. childish
   - B. mature
   - C. feverish
   - D. immaculate
   - E. pusillanimous

   2.____

3. PUNCTILIOUS
   - A. offensively frank
   - B. willing to admit blame
   - C. sarcastically polite
   - D. precise in conduct
   - E. indiscriminate

   3.____

4. RAZE
   - A. torture
   - B. erect
   - C. salvage
   - D. destroy
   - E. prorogue

   4.____

5. RECESSIVE
   - A. inclined to go back
   - B. relating to slavery
   - C. moving forward
   - D. modest
   - E. allemorphic

   5.____

6. RENEGADE
   - A. turncoat
   - B. loyalist
   - C. habitual drunkard
   - D. confirmed criminal
   - E. one who kills a king

   6.____

7. RENASCENCE
   - A. unwinding
   - B. restoration
   - C. unscrewing
   - D. detraining
   - E. perdition

   7.____

8. RESPITE
   - A. pardon
   - B. re-trial
   - C. stay
   - D. vengeance
   - E. continuation

   8.____

9. SALIENT
   - A. hidden
   - B. salty
   - C. floating
   - D. prominent
   - E. flagrant

   9.____

10. SATELLITE
    - A. falling star
    - B. attentive follower
    - C. adversary
    - D. flint spark
    - E. fellow captive

    10.____

11. SCRUPULOUS   11.____

    A. niggardly   B. abusive   C. conscientious
    D. unprincipled   E. guilty

12. SINEWY   12.____

    A. callused   B. enervated   C. springy
    D. slimy   E. brawny

13. SKEPTIC   13.____

    A. agnostic   B. suave   C. ingenious
    D. credulous   E. faithful

14. SPARE   14.____

    A. forbear   B. forego   C. reserve
    D. control   E. squander

15. SPORADIC   15.____

    A. isolated   B. incessant   C. dissipated
    D. involuntary   E. discrete

KEYS (CORRECT ANSWERS)

1. E   6. B
2. B   7. E
3. E   8. E
4. B   9. A
5. C   10. C

11. D
12. B
13. D
14. E
15. B

ANTONYMS/OPPOSITES

EXAMINATION SECTION
TEST 1

DIRECTIONS: Each question below consists of a word printed in capital letters, followed by five words or phrases lettered A through E. Choose the lettered word or phrase that is MOST NEARLY OPPOSITE in meaning to the word in capital letters. *PRINT THE LETTER OF THE CORRECT ANSWER IN THE SPACE AT THE RIGHT.*

1. QUALIFIED

    A. tight
    D. serene
    B. unfit
    E. necessary
    C. chosen

    1._____

2. IMMATERIAL

    A. radial
    D. diffuse
    B. tangible
    E. unproved
    C. minute

    2._____

3. THRIVE

    A. terminate
    D. enjoy
    B. swell
    E. strive
    C. languish

    3._____

4. UNDERTAKE

    A. refrain
    D. identify
    B. conceal
    E. address
    C. decide

    4._____

5. REMOVABLE

    A. indelible
    D. uncommon
    B. threadbare
    E. fictitious
    C. legible

    5._____

6. PRIOR

    A. primary
    D. subsequent
    B. contemporary
    E. simultaneous
    C. recent

    6._____

7. YIELDING

    A. unsympathetic
    D. adamant
    B. moist
    E. pressing
    C. modern

    7._____

8. ABYSS

    A. buttress
    D. surface
    B. hinge
    E. oblivion
    C. pinnacle

    8._____

9. MOURN

    A. commemorate
    D. deny
    B. welcome
    E. exult
    C. change

    9._____

10. ABUSE

    A. plaudit
    D. insight
    B. indecisiveness
    E. silence
    C. elegance

    10._____

11. UNION
    A. majority   B. schism   C. uniformity
    D. conference E. construction

12. SUBMISSIVE
    A. dense   B. refractory   C. polite
    D. stable   E. concentrating

13. OBJECT OF DERISION
    A. emetic   B. stimulant   C. paragon
    D. scapegoat E. mendicant

14. AVERSION
    A. foible   B. flagrant   C. weakness
    D. penchant E. mischance

15. GAY
    A. nagging   B. exuberant   C. triumphant
    D. howling   E. plaintive

16. REVEAL IN TRUE FORM
    A. see through   B. imitate   C. express
    D. dissimulate   E. invade

17. ACCLAIM
    A. aid   B. express condolence   C. excoriate
    D. cover   E. clothe

18. PASSED AWAY
    A. sick   B. moribund   C. extant
    D. near   E. remote

19. UNDERSTATEMENT
    A. exact statement   B. restraint   C. high spirits
    D. hyperbole   E. low spirits

20. SULLIED
    A. inviolable   B. dishonorable   C. invidious
    D. public   E. commonplace

21. HEALTHFUL
    A. noxious   B. balmy   C. healthy
    D. nubile   E. salubrious

22. ORDER
    A. panic   B. rigidity   C. indolence
    D. innocence E. discipline

23. PLENTY

    A. vastness   B. paucity   C. mass
    D. regiment   E. number

24. BESEECHING

    A. pleasant   B. calm   C. peremptory
    D. inviting   E. carping

25. EARNEST MANNER

    A. banal   B. harsh manner   C. persiflage
    D. wisdom   E. sorrow

KEY (CORRECT ANSWERS)

1.	B	11.	B
2.	B	12.	B
3.	C	13.	C
4.	A	14.	D
5.	A	15.	E
6.	D	16.	D
7.	D	17.	C
8.	C	18.	C
9.	E	19.	D
10.	A	20.	A

21. A
22. A
23. B
24. C
25. C

TEST 2

DIRECTIONS: Each question below consists of a word printed in capital letters, followed by five words or phrases lettered A through E. Choose the lettered word or phrase that is MOST NEARLY OPPOSITE in meaning to the word in capital letters. *PRINT THE LETTER OF THE CORRECT ANSWER IN THE SPACE AT THE RIGHT.*

1. PATENT 1.____
   - A. obvious
   - B. hidden
   - C. equivocal
   - D. frank
   - E. wilful

2. ENRAGE 2.____
   - A. support
   - B. be angry
   - C. yield
   - D. mollify
   - E. torment

3. SOFT SPOKEN 3.____
   - A. smear
   - B. polite
   - C. raucous
   - D. noxious
   - E. mending

4. ABUNDANCE 4.____
   - A. riches
   - B. magnanimity
   - C. sufficient
   - D. paucity
   - E. abbreviation

5. BENEFICIAL 5.____
   - A. inserted
   - B. prosperous
   - C. benign
   - D. deleterious
   - E. missionary

6. SUBJECT OF AVERSION 6.____
   - A. trustful
   - B. cynosure
   - C. subject of ridicule
   - D. evil omen
   - E. iniquitous

7. INTRANSIGENT 7.____
   - A. resentful
   - B. negative
   - C. be determined
   - D. acquiescent
   - E. unruly

8. WASTREL 8.____
   - A. prodigious
   - B. costly
   - C. luxurious
   - D. prodigal
   - E. parsimonious

9. LAPSE OF MEMORY 9.____
   - A. forgetful
   - B. thoughtless
   - C. incentive
   - D. recollection
   - E. induction

10. PERSPICACIOUS 10.____
    - A. erudite
    - B. dull
    - C. tactful
    - D. persistent
    - E. mandatory

11. RECONDITE 11.____
    - A. mumbling
    - B. poorly defined
    - C. concise
    - D. abstract
    - E. grandiloquent

2 (#2)

12. ELEMENTARY 12._____
    A. famous B. alimentary C. popular
    D. ambiguous E. pristine

13. IN PERSON 13._____
    A. normal B. genuine C. vicarious
    D. original E. legendary

14. REDOLENT 14._____
    A. malodorous B. fragrant C. aromatic
    D. odor of cooking E. redundant

15. REPELLING 15._____
    A. shy B. diffident C. contemptible
    D. prepossessing E. rebelling

16. DIRECT 16._____
    A. using subterfuge B. naive C. covenant
    D. guide E. express

17. SERIOUS 17._____
    A. facetious B. dull C. stern
    D. uninteresting E. loathsome

18. REALITY 18._____
    A. illusion B. image C. sanity
    D. panic E. caution

19. ENERGETIC 19._____
    A. prompt B. cordial C. enervated
    D. effusive E. meandering

20. LETHARGIC 20._____
    A. dormant B. nimble C. tardy
    D. baronial E. lissome

21. DISPUTABLE 21._____
    A. untrue B. incontrovertible C. unproven
    D. uncertain E. recondite

22. ANCHORITE 22._____
    A. gregarious B. lonely C. hostile
    D. alien E. privately

23. GOOD LUCK 23._____
    A. calm B. peace C. drought
    D. cataclysm E. fortuitous

24. AVARICE

    A. generosity   B. wastefulness   C. kindness
    D. self-seeking   E. covetousness

24.____

25. UNYIELDING

    A. passive   B. obedient   C. tractable
    D. adamant   E. intractable

25.____

KEY (CORRECT ANSWERS)

1.	C	11.	C
2.	D	12.	D
3.	C	13.	C
4.	D	14.	A
5.	D	15.	D
6.	B	16.	A
7.	D	17.	A
8.	E	18.	A
9.	D	19.	C
10.	B	20.	B

21. B
22. A
23. D
24. A
25. C

TEST 3

DIRECTIONS: Each question below consists of a word printed in capital letters, followed by five words or phrases lettered A through E. Choose the lettered word or phrase that is MOST NEARLY OPPOSITE in meaning to the word in capital letters. *PRINT THE LETTER OF THE CORRECT ANSWER IN THE SPACE AT THE RIGHT.*

1. SUBSEQUENT
    - A. symbolic
    - B. reserved
    - C. unjust
    - D. preceding
    - E. following

2. REPLETE
    - A. true
    - B. wanting
    - C. grim
    - D. drab
    - E. greedy

3. INSINCERE
    - A. treacherous
    - B. unfeigned
    - C. opaque
    - D. rnaroon
    - E. helpful

4. FRAUDULENT
    - A. honest
    - B. dishonest
    - C. pathetic
    - D. greedy
    - E. dry

5. ARTLESSNESS
    - A. affectation
    - B. fidelity
    - C. guiltlessness
    - D. probity
    - E. truthfulness

6. IMMODERATE
    - A. modest
    - B. temperate
    - C. obscene
    - D. fretful
    - E. grumpy

7. ATROCIOUSNESS
    - A. stinginess
    - B. inhumanity
    - C. harshness
    - D. barbarity
    - E. kindness

8. ATTRACTION
    - A. coveting
    - B. aversion
    - C. fancy
    - D. longing
    - E. lust

9. ASININE
    - A. empty
    - B. cloddish
    - C. clever
    - D. bungling
    - E. driveling

10. ASPERSION
    - A. praise
    - B. disapprobation
    - C. discredit
    - D. blame
    - E. jeers

1. _____
2. _____
3. _____
4. _____
5. _____
6. _____
7. _____
8. _____
9. _____
10. _____

KEY (CORRECT ANSWERS)

1. D
2. B
3. B
4. A
5. A
6. B
7. E
8. B
9. C
10. A

TEST 4

DIRECTIONS: Each question below consists of a word printed in capital letters, followed by five words or phrases lettered A through E. Choose the lettered word or phrase that is MOST NEARLY OPPOSITE in meaning to the word in capital letters. *PRINT THE LETTER OF THE CORRECT ANSWER IN THE SPACE AT THE RIGHT.*

1. CAUSTIC
   - A. mild
   - B. harsh
   - C. gritty
   - D. greasy
   - E. raw

   1.____

2. BIGOTED
   - A. hateful
   - B. ignorant
   - C. subtle
   - D. tolerant
   - E. alert

   2.____

3. FINICAL
   - A. fastidious
   - B. attractive
   - C. happy
   - D. filthy
   - E. leafy

   3.____

4. REFRESHED
   - A. crisp
   - B. joyous
   - C. fatigued
   - D. mute
   - E. sickly

   4.____

5. CRAFTY
   - A. watchful
   - B. creative
   - C. candid
   - D. ignoble
   - E. shy

   5.____

6. ASSIDUOUS
   - A. quick
   - B. keen
   - C. energetic
   - D. active
   - E. phlegmatic

   6.____

7. ASSIST
   - A. clarify
   - B. expound
   - C. cramp
   - D. promote
   - E. untangle

   7.____

8. ASSURANCE
   - A. credence
   - B. conviction
   - C. certainty
   - D. reliance
   - E. doubt

   8.____

9. AT A LOW EBB
   - A. fewer
   - B. above
   - C. under
   - D. less
   - E. below

   9.____

10. AT NO TIME
    - A. always
    - B. never
    - C. on no occasion
    - D. nevermore
    - E. momentarily

    10.____

KEY (CORRECT ANSWERS)

1. A
2. D
3. D
4. C
5. C

11. E
12. C
13. E
14. B
15. A

SAME-OPPOSITE (SYNONYM-ANTONYM) EXAMINATION SECTION

TEST 1

DIRECTIONS: Each question in this part consists of a word printed in capital letters followed by five words lettered A through E. Choose the letter of the word that is most nearly the SAME in meaning OR the OPPOSITE of the word in capital letters. *PRINT THE LETTER OF THE CORRECT ANSWER IN THE SPACE AT THE RIGHT.*

1. FURTIVE
   A. strong
   B. colorless
   C. listless
   D. serene
   E. stealthy

2. UNDAUNTED
   A. thick
   B. abrupt
   C. intrepid
   D. valid
   E. reserved

3. BESEECHING
   A. inviting
   B. carping
   C. peremptory
   D. calm
   E. pleasant

4. ABYSS
   A. surface
   B. amiss
   C. pinnacle
   D. hinge
   E. buttress

5. SUBMISSIVE
   A. stable
   B. polite
   C. refractory
   D. dense
   E. concentrating

6. HURTLE
   A. hurdle
   B. trip
   C. rush headlong
   D. jump over
   E. throw out

7. UNYIELDING
   A. prehensile
   B. adipose
   C. tractable
   D. panicky
   E. impartial

8. AUGMENT
   A. promise
   B. urge
   C. dispute
   D. arrange
   E. increase

9. TORPID
   A. fat
   B. tepid
   C. hot
   D. lukewarm
   E. sluggish

10. PROPENSITY
    A. kindliness
    B. proprietary
    C. feebleness
    D. agility
    E. tendency

11. CALUMNIATE
    A. advance	B. slander	C. shameful
    D. conspire	E. paint
    11._____

12. ABUSE
    A. plaudit	B. elegance	C. silence
    D. insight	E. collation
    12._____

13. SULLIED
    A. inviolable	B. common	C. unhampered
    D. invidious	E. neat
    13._____

14. ANCHORITIC
    A. like a stone		B. authoritarian
    C. pertaining to an anchor	D. disputatious
    E. gregarious
    14._____

15. MOURN
    A. measure	B. meander	C. change
    D. exit	E. deny
    15._____

16. MOTLEY
    A. realistic	B. remote	C. rugged
    D. mixed	E. hardy
    16._____

17. IMMATERIAL
    A. diffuse	B. tangible	C. minute
    D. migrant	E. unilateral
    17._____

18. PAUCITY
    A. magnanimity	B. sufficient	C. abbreviation
    D. abundance	E. mitigation
    18._____

19. BLITHE
    A. rosy	B. pastoral	C. dusty
    D. bland	E. cheerful
    19._____

20. RIBALD
    A. coarse	B. shrunken	C. laughing
    D. sinister	E. balding
    20._____

21. SERIOUS
    A. facetious	B. dull	C. limpid
    D. uninteresting	E. loathsome
    21._____

22. REALITY
    A. sanity	B. panic	C. illusion
    D. hope	E. caution
    22._____

23. EMBLEMATIC
   A. supreme   B. hospitable   C. unjust
   D. symbolic   E. balmy

24. HEALTHFUL
   A. billowy   B. true   C. salubrious
   D. stubborn   E. connubial

25. TREMULOUS
   A. loud   B. quavering   C. leafy
   D. girlish   E. pristine

KEY (CORRECT ANSWERS)

1.	E (S)		11.	B (S)
2.	C (S)		12.	A (O)
3.	C (O)		13.	A (O)
4.	C (O)		14.	E (O)
5.	C (O)		15.	D (O)
6.	C (S)		16.	D (S)
7.	C (O)		17.	B (O)
8.	E (S)		18.	D (O)
9.	E (S)		19.	E (S)
10.	E (S)		20.	A (S)

21.	A (O)
22.	C (O)
23.	D (S)
24.	C (S)
25.	B (S)

TEST 2

DIRECTIONS: Each question in this part consists of a word printed in capital letters followed by five words lettered A through E. Choose the letter of the word that is most nearly the SAME in meaning OR the OPPOSITE of the word in capital letters. *PRINT THE LETTER OF THE CORRECT ANSWER IN THE SPACE AT THE RIGHT.*

1. VIXEN
   A. virus
   B. shrewd person
   C. termagant
   D. thief
   E. snake

2. DISCURSIVE
   A. rambling
   B. discreet
   C. evasive
   D. disgusting
   E. absurd

3. VERACIOUS
   A. begging
   B. mendacious
   C. avaricious
   D. voracious
   E. perspicacious

4. DENIZEN
   A. a citizen
   B. a wild beast
   C. a dweller
   D. a savage
   E. a hermit

5. FRUGAL
   A. fertile
   B. giant
   C. prodigal
   D. tiny
   E. minimal

6. PLAUSIBLE
   A. firm
   B. fiction
   C. specious
   D. praiseworthy
   E. amenable

7. DOLEFUL
   A. extemporary
   B. extant
   C. egregious
   D. jocular
   E. exemplary

8. TETE-A-TETE
   A. girlfriend
   B. flirt
   C. alliance
   D. confidential chat
   E. testy

9. EMOLLIENT
   A. greasy
   B. miserly
   C. soothing
   D. tactful
   E. rewarding

10. EXTRANEOUS
    A. sapient
    B. inebriated
    C. intrinsic
    D. incipient
    E. gasping

2 (#2)

11. PATENT
    A. mixing   B. originating   C. lingering
    D. latent   E. nascent
    11.____

12. CHIDE
    A. expurgate   B. reprove   C. rejoin
    D. defile   E. cherish
    12.____

13. FORMIDABLE
    A. serried   B. magical   C. technical
    D. menacing   E. troublesome
    13.____

14. CONCUPISCENCE
    A. wisdom   B. conspiracy   C. jealousy
    D. lust   E. eagerness
    14.____

15. FELINE
    A. cat-like   B. slim   C. dainty
    D. feminine   E. criminal
    15.____

16. INDIGENT
    A. native   B. inherent   C. opulent
    D. digestible   E. indecent
    16.____

17. EVENTUATE
    A. to plan   B. to come to pass   C. to experience
    D. to vanish   E. to pass away
    17.____

18. DEMAND
    A. to prevent   B. exult   C. inveigh
    D. implore   E. deter
    18.____

19. CONDONE
    A. integrate   B. imprecate   C. convey
    D. exonerate   E. delude
    19.____

20. IMPROPRIETY
    A. decoration   B. sobriety   C. seemliness
    D. timidity   E. misappropriation
    20.____

21. VILLAINOUS
    A. rascally   B. optic   C. subtle
    D. wiry   E. rustic
    21.____

22. AVARICIOUS
    A. dirty   B. oily   C. obnoxious
    D. greedy   E. averse
    22.____

23. FLAGRANT
    A. complacent   B. egregious   C. ephemeral
    D. fiery   E. flag-waving

24. ASPERITY
    A. matrimony   B. acrimony   C. ceremony
    D. testimony   E. alimony

25. PEREMPTORY
    A. pertinent   B. indecisive   C. marketable
    D. pathetic   E. permissible

KEY (CORRECT ANSWERS)

1.	C (S)		11.	D (O)
2.	A (S)		12.	B (O)
3.	B (O)		13.	D (S)
4.	C (S)		14.	D (S)
5.	C (O)		15.	A (S)
6.	C (O)		16.	C (O)
7.	D (O)		17.	B (S)
8.	D (S)		18.	D (O)
9.	C (S)		19.	D (S)
10.	C (O)		20.	C (O)

21. A (S)
22. D (S)
23. B (S)
24. B (S)
25. B (O)

TEST 3

DIRECTIONS: Each question in this part consists of a word printed in capital letters followed by five words lettered A through E. Choose the letter of the word that is most nearly the SAME in meaning OR the OPPOSITE of the word in capital letters. *PRINT THE LETTER OF THE CORRECT ANSWER IN THE SPACE AT THE RIGHT.*

1. AUSPICIOUS
   A. malicious   B. popular   C. awesome
   D. suspicious   E. propitious

   1.____

2. PETULANT
   A. amiable   B. religious   C. penitent
   D. petty   E. pesty

   2.____

3. MARTIAL
   A. miraculous   B. highest military rank   C. pacific
   D. maritime   E. marital

   3.____

4. FAIN
   A. feign   B. inimical   C. reverse
   D. divided   E. found

   4.____

5. ELICIT
   A. solicit   B. implicit   C. conducive
   D. exhibit   E. exact

   5.____

6. CONTEMPTIBLE
   A. indomitable   B. despicable   C. reversible
   D. comtemporary   E. temporary

   6.____

7. ADAMANT
   A. vacillating   B. vacuous   C. osculate
   D. clamorous   E. sedimentary

   7.____

8. FEIGN
   A. resemble   B. assemble   C. ensemble
   D. tremble   E. dissemble

   8.____

9. ANTICIPATE
   A. gather   B. recollect   C. resign
   D. undermine   E. pander

   9.____

10. AMBIGUOUS
    A. equivocal   B. awry   C. bigoted
    D. ambulatory   E. generic

    10.____

247

11. PERMIT
    A. launder   B. ponder   C. enjoin
    D. reveal   E. grimace
    11.____

12. OMNISCIENT
    A. permissive   B. obtuse   C. offensive
    D. reminiscent E. ravishing
    12.____

13. MUTE
    A. petite   B. speechless   C. mite
    D. mighty   E. lackadaisical
    13.____

14. QUALIFIED
    A. tight   B. incompetent   C. chosen
    D. necessary   E. serene
    14.____

15. LACONIC
    A. fertile   B. recalcitrant   C. penurious
    D. rigid   E. pithy
    15.____

16. BELLIGERENT
    A. urban   B. endemic   C. condign
    D. reserved   E. peaceful
    16.____

17. RELENTLESS
    A. secure   B. severe   C. intractable
    D. sincere   E. boring
    17.____

18. ANTIPATHY
    A. pathology   B. goodwill   C. burden
    D. status   E. coupon
    18.____

19. AUTHENTIC
    A. arid   B. avid   C. actual
    D. auxiliary   E. antiquated
    19.____

20. DIFFIDENT
    A. faithful   B. confident   C. arrogant
    D. concealed   E. involved
    20.____

21. PROLIXITY
    A. erectness   B. mastery   C. succinctness
    D. sapidity   E. ferocity
    21.____

22. HEDONIST
    A. prohibitionist   B. regionalist   C. atheist
    D. conformist   E. ascetic
    22.____

23. DEPRECATE
    A. depreciate B. dessicate C. approve
    D. abbreviate E. condone

    23.____

24. ANTAGONISTIC
    A. macabre B. regional C. amicable
    D. salutary E. materialistic

    24.____

25. REMOTE
    A. garish B. artificial C. contiguous
    D. reaching E. remiss

    25.____

KEY (CORRECT ANSWERS)

1.	E (S)		11.	C (O)
2.	A (O)		12.	B (O)
3.	C (O)		13.	B (S)
4.	B (O)		14.	B (O)
5.	E (S)		15.	E (S)
6.	B (S)		16.	E (O)
7.	A (O)		17.	C (O)
8.	E (S)		18.	B (O)
9.	B (O)		19.	C (S)
10.	A (S)		20.	B (O)

21. C (O)
22. E (O)
23. C (O)
24. C (O)
25. C (O)

TEST 4

DIRECTIONS: Each question in this part consists of a word printed in capital letters followed by five words lettered A through E. Choose the letter of the word that is most nearly the SAME in meaning OR the OPPOSITE of the word in capital letters. *PRINT THE LETTER OF THE CORRECT ANSWER IN THE SPACE AT THE RIGHT.*

1. MAGNANIMOUS
   A. earthy
   B. ghastly
   C. sinister
   D. churlish
   E. pelagic

   1.____

2. DEFTNESS
   A. skill
   B. complacency
   C. transition
   D. acuity
   E. protocol

   2.____

3. HEINOUS
   A. extinct
   B. thoughtful
   C. monstrous
   D. highest
   E. hirsute

   3.____

4. PERSPICUOUS
   A. conspicuous
   B. obscure
   C. scanty
   D. tiring
   E. curvaceous

   4.____

5. PROSELYTIZE
   A. allege
   B. publicize
   C. convert
   D. compel
   E. promulgate

   5.____

6. DEFORM
   A. inform
   B. perform
   C. conform
   D. change
   E. embellish

   6.____

7. EMULATE
   A. emanate
   B. rival
   C. coordinate
   D. infiltrate
   E. coagulate

   7.____

8. DILATE
   A. contract
   B. dilute
   C. expire
   D. retain
   E. collate

   8.____

9. INDOCTRINATE
   A. unlearn
   B. collaborate
   C. substitute
   D. reveal
   E. marinate

   9.____

10. ACME
    A. efflorescent
    B. magic
    C. reaction
    D. pimple
    E. nadir

    10.____

2 (#4)

11. INCISIVE
    A. talkative   B. arrant   C. basic
    D. trenchant   E. motley
    11.____

12. PUSILLANIMITY
    A. pertaining to pus   B. potentiality   C. hauteur
    D. sterility   E. valor
    12.____

13. PALLID
    A. nasty   B. covering   C. callow
    D. vivid   E. incandescent
    13.____

14. TURGID
    A. tumid   B. humid   C. fuming
    D. regurgitate   E. frigid
    14.____

15. TEMERITY
    A. celerity   B. brevity   C. audacity
    D. arduousness   E. majesty
    15.____

16. AFFLUENT
    A. fluent   B. fluid   C. frugal
    D. mendacious   E. impecunious
    16.____

17. REDUNDANT
    A. bountiful   B. agile   C. repetitive
    D. occasional   E. mordant
    17.____

18. INTENSIFY
    A. convince   B. abate   C. seduce
    D. abet   E. ferret
    18.____

19. REBUKE
    A. administer   B. retire   C. eulogize
    D. acquiesce   E. render
    19.____

20. VICARIOUS
    A. pertaining to the vicarage   B. slanderous
    C. viperous   D. direct
    E. measure of area
    20.____

21. TANGIBLE
    A. pertaining to a tangent   B. tandem   C. substantial
    D. substitutionary   E. miasmic
    21.____

22. PUERILE
    A. mature   B. simian   C. parrot-like
    D. passive   E. malodorous
    22.____

23. CONTEMPORARY
   A. temporary
   B. contemptuous
   C. accessory
   D. pristine
   E. creative

23.____

24. INHIBIT
   A. undervalue
   B. relax
   C. unruly
   D. magnify
   E. impede

24.____

25. VALID
   A. sallow
   B. efficacious
   C. marginal
   D. candid
   E. valorous

25.____

KEY (CORRECT ANSWERS)

1. D (O)
2. A (S)
3. C (S)
4. B (O)
5. C (S)

6. E (O)
7. B (S)
8. A (O)
9. A (O)
10. E (O)

11. D (S)
12. E (O)
13. D (O)
14. A (S)
15. C (S)

16. E (O)
17. C (S)
18. B (O)
19. C (O)
20. D (O)

21. C (S)
22. A (O)
23. D (O)
24. E (S)
25. B (S)

TEST 5

DIRECTIONS: Each question in this part consists of a word printed in capital letters followed by five words lettered A through E. Choose the letter of the word that is most nearly the SAME in meaning OR the OPPOSITE of the word in capital letters. *PRINT THE LETTER OF THE CORRECT ANSWER IN THE SPACE AT THE RIGHT.*

1. SEDULOUS
   A. trusting
   B. lax
   C. expanded
   D. serving
   E. satiny

   1.____

2. ENCOMIUM
   A. pertaining to opium
   B. obloquy
   C. greeting
   D. victory
   E. unit

   2.____

3. EXTRAORDINARY
   A. creative
   B. emotional
   C. sorry
   D. flighty
   E. egregious

   3.____

4. REDOLENT
   A. tasty
   B. rude
   C. threatening
   D. odorous
   E. beginning

   4.____

5. IMMINENT
   A. eminent
   B. stupendous
   C. imposing
   D. reducing
   E. impending

   5.____

6. SANG-FROID
   A. miserliness
   B. tenacity
   C. brutality
   D. fearfulness
   E. petulance

   6.____

7. TRUCULENT
   A. frightful
   B. terrific
   C. placid
   D. tricky
   E. sycophantic

   7.____

8. PREVARICATION
   A. honest
   B. generosity
   C. veracity
   D. variation
   E. differentiation

   8.____

9. INCORPOREAL
   A. brusque
   B. happy
   C. troubled
   D. carping
   E. immaterial

   9.____

10. TENUOUS
    A. accurate
    B. flabby
    C. thin
    D. temporary
    E. tendentious

    10.____

253

11. NUANCE
    A. hint
    B. subtle difference
    C. trickery
    D. modesty
    E. stance

    11.____

12. TEMPORAL
    A. tempting
    B. tangible
    C. memorizing
    D. peculiar
    E. spiritual

    12.____

KEY (CORRECT ANSWERS)

1. B (O)
2. B (O)
3. E (S)
4. D (S)
5. E (S)
6. D (O)
7. C (O)
8. C (O)
9. E (S)
10. C (S)
11. B (S)
12. E (O)

TESTS IN SENTENCE COMPLETION / 1 BLANK
EXAMINATION SECTION
TEST 1

DIRECTIONS: Each question in this section consists of a sentence in which one word is missing; a blank line indicates where the word has been removed from the sentence. Beneath each sentence are five words, *one* of which is the missing word. You are to select the letter of the missing word by deciding which one of the five words BEST fits in with the meaning of the sentence. *PRINT THE LETTER OF THE CORRECT ANSWER IN THE SPACE AT THE RIGHT.*

1. A man who cannot win honor in his own _____ will have a very small chance of winning it from posterity.

   A. right   B. field   C. country   D. way   E. age

2. The latent period for the contractile response to direct stimulation of the muscle has quite another and shorte value, encompassing only a utilization period. Hence it is that the term *latent period* must be _____ carefully each time that it is used.

   A. checked   B. timed   C. introduced
   D. defined   E. selected

3. Many television watchers enjoy stories which contain violence. Consequently those television producers who are dominated by rating systems aim to _____ the popular taste.

   A. raise   B. control   C. gratify   D. ignore   E. lower

4. No other man loses so much, so _____, so absolutely, as the beaten candidate for high public office.

   A. bewilderingly   B. predictably   C. disgracefully
   D. publicly   E. cheerfully

5. Mathematics is the product of thought operating by means of _____ for the purpose of expressing general laws.

   A. reasoning   B. symbols   C. words
   D. examples   E. science

6. Deductive reasoning is that form of reasoning in which the conclusion must necessarily follow if we accept the premise as true. In deduction, it is _____ the premise to be true and the conclusion false.

   A. impossible   B. inevitable   C. reasonable
   D. surprising   E. unlikely

7. Because in the administration it hath respect not to the group but to the _____, our form of government is called a democracy.

   A. courts   B. people   C. majority
   D. individual   E. law

8. Before criticizing the work of an artist one needs to _____ the artist's purpose.

   A. understand   B. reveal   C. defend
   D. correct   E. change

9. Their work was commemorative in character and consisted largely of _____ erected upon the occasion of victories.

   A. towers   B. tombs   C. monuments
   D. castles   E. fortresses

10. Every good story is carefully contrived: the elements of the story are _____ to fit with one another in order to make an effect on the reader.

    A. read   B. learned   C. emphasized
    D. reduced   E. planned

KEY (CORRECT ANSWERS)

1. E	6. A
2. D	7. D
3. C	8. A
4. D	9. C
5. B	10. E

TEST 2

DIRECTIONS: Each question in this section consists of a sentence in which one word is missing; a blank line indicates where the word has been removed from the sentence. Beneath each sentence are five words, *one* of which is the missing word. You are to select the letter of the missing word by deciding which one of the five words BEST fits in with the meaning of the sentence. *PRINT THE LETTER OF THE CORRECT ANSWER IN THE SPACE AT THE RIGHT.*

1. One of the most prevalent erroneous contentions is that Argentina is a country of _____ agricultural resources and needs only the arrival of ambitious settlers.

    A. modernized B. flourishing C. undeveloped
    D. waning E. limited

    1.____

2. The last official statistics for the town indicated the presence of 24,212 Italians, 6,450 Magyars, and 2,315 Germans, which ensures to the _____ a numerical preponderance.

    A. Germans B. figures C. town D. Magyars E. Italians

    2.____

3. Precision of wording is necessary in good writing; by choosing words that exactly convey the desired meaning, one can avoid _____.

    A. duplicity B. incongruity C. complexity
    D. ambiguity E. implications

    3.____

4. Various civilians of the liberal school in the British Parliament remonstrated that there were no grounds for _____ of French aggression, since the Emperor showed less disposition to augment the navy than had Louis Philippe.

    A. suppression B. retaliation C. apprehension
    D. concealment E. commencement

    4.____

5. _____ is as clear and definite as any of our urges; we wonder what is in a sealed letter or what is being said in a telephone booth.

    A. Envy B. Curiosity C. Knowledge
    D. Communication E. Ambition

    5.____

6. It is a rarely philosophic soul who can make a _____ the other alternative forever into the limbo of forgotten things.

    A. mistake B. wish C. change D. choice E. plan

    6.____

7. A creditor is worse than a master. A master owns only your person, but a creditor owns your _____ as well.

    A. aspirations B. potentialities C. ideas
    D. dignity E. wealth

    7.____

8. People _____ small faults, in order to insinuate that they have no great ones.

    A. create B. display C. confess D. seek E. reject

    8.____

9. Andrew Jackson believed that wars were inevitable, and to him the length and irregularity of our coast presented a _____ that called for a more than merely passive navy.

   A. defense
   B. barrier
   C. provocation
   D. vulnerability
   E. dispute

10. The progressive yearly _____ of the land, caused by the depositing of mud from the river, makes it possible to estimate the age of excavated remains by noting the depth at which they are found below the present level of the valley.

    A. erosion
    B. elevation
    C. improvement
    D. irrigation
    E. displacement

KEY (CORRECT ANSWERS)

1. C
2. E
3. D
4. C
5. B
6. D
7. D
8. C
9. D
10. B

TEST 3

DIRECTIONS: Each question in this section consists of a sentence in which one word is missing; a blank line indicates where the word has been removed from the sentence. Beneath each sentence are five words, *one* of which is the missing word. You are to select the letter of the missing word by deciding which one of the five words BEST fits in with the meaning of the sentence. *PRINT THE LETTER OF THE CORRECT ANSWER IN THE SPACE AT THE RIGHT.*

1. The judge exercised commendable _____ dismissing the charge against the prisoner. In spite of the clamor that surrounded the trial, and the heinousness of the offense, the judge could not be swayed to overlook the lack of facts in the case.

    A. avidity B. meticulousness C. clemency
    D. balance E. querulousness

    1.____

2. The pianist played the concerto _____, displaying such facility and skill as has rarely been matched in this old auditorium.

    A. strenuous B. spiritedly C. passionately
    D. casually E. deftly

    2.____

3. The Tanglewood Symphony Orchestra holds its outdoor concerts far from city turmoil in a _____, bucolic setting.

    A. spectacular B. atavistic C. serene
    D. chaotic E. catholic

    3.____

4. Honest satire gives true joy to the thinking man. Thus, the satirist is most _____ when he points out the hypocrisy in human actions.

    A. elated B. humiliated C. ungainly
    D. repressed E. disdainful

    4.____

5. She was a(n) _____ preferred the company of her books to the pleasures of cafe society.

    A. philanthropist B. stoic C. exhibitionist
    D. extrovert E. introvert

    5.____

6. So many people are so convinced that people are driven by _____ motives that they cannot believe that anybody is unselfish!

    A. interior B. ulterior C. unworth
    D. selfish E. destructive

    6.____

7. These _____ results were brought about by a chain of fortuitous events.

    A. unfortunate B. odd C. harmful
    D. haphazard E. propitious

    7.____

8. The bank teller's _____ of the funds was discovered the following month when the auditors examined the books.

    A. embezzlement B. burglary C. borrowing
    D. assignment E. theft

    8.____

259

9. The monks gathered in the _____ for their evening meal.   9._____

    A. lounge   B. auditorium   C. refectory
    D. rectory   E. solarium

10. Local officials usually have the responsibility in each area of determining when the need   10._____
    is sufficiently great to _____ withdrawals from the community water supply.

    A. encourage   B. justify   C. discontinue
    D. advocate   E. forbid

KEY (CORRECT ANSWERS)

1. D   6. B
2. E   7. D
3. C   8. A
4. A   9. C
5. E   10. B

TEST 4

DIRECTIONS: Each question in this section consists of a sentence in which one word is missing; a blank line indicates where the word has been removed from the sentence. Beneath each sentence are five words, *one* of which is the missing word. You are to select the letter of the missing word by deciding which one of the five words BEST fits in with the meaning of the sentence. *PRINT THE LETTER OF THE CORRECT ANSWER IN THE SPACE AT THE RIGHT*

1. The life of the mining camps as portrayed by Bret Harte–boisterous, material, brawling– was in direct _____ to the contemporary Eastern world of conventional morals and staid deportment depicted by other men of letters.

    A. model B. parallel C. antithesis
    D. relationship E. response

2. The agreements were to remain in force for three years and were subject to automatic _____ unless terminated by the parties concerned on one month's notice.

    A. renewal B. abrogation C. amendment
    D. confiscation E. option

3. In a democracy, people are recognized for what they do rather than for their _____.

    A. alacrity B. ability C. reputation
    D. skill E. pedigree

4. Although he had often loudly proclaimed his _____ concerning world affairs, he actually read widely and was usually the best informed person in his circle.

    A. weariness B. complacency C. condolence
    D. indifference E. worry

5. This student holds the _____ record of being the sole failure in his class.

    A. flagrant B. unhappy C. egregious
    D. dubious E. unusual

6. She became enamored _____ acrobat when she witnessed his act.

    A. of B. with C. for D. by E. about

7. This will _____ all previous wills.

    A. abrogates B. denies C. supersedes
    D. prevents E. continues

8. In the recent terrible Chicago _____, over ninety children were found dead as a result of the fire.

    A. hurricane B. destruction C. panic
    D. holocaust E. accident

9. I can ascribe no better reason why he shunned society than that he was a _____.

    A. mentor B. Centaur C. aristocrat
    D. misanthrope E. failure

10. One who attempts to learn all the known facts before he comes to a conclusion may most aptly be described as a _____.

   A. realist
   B. philosopher
   C. cynic
   D. pessimist
   E. skeptic

KEY (CORRECT ANSWERS)

1. C
2. A
3. E
4. D
5. D
6. A
7. C
8. D
9. D
10. E

TEST 5

DIRECTIONS: Each question in this section consists of a sentence in which one word is missing; a blank line indicates where the word has been removed from the sentence. Beneath each sentence are five words, *one* of which is the missing word. You are to select the letter of the missing word by deciding which one of the five words BEST fits in with the meaning of the sentence. *PRINT THE LETTER OF THE CORRECT ANSWER IN THE SPACE AT THE RIGHT.*

1. The prime minister, fleeing from the rebels who had seized the government, sought _____ in the church.

   A. revenge B. mercy C. relief
   D. salvation E. sanctuary

   1.____

2. It does not take us long to conclude that it is foolish to fight the _____, and that it is far wiser to accept it.

   A. inevitable B. inconsequential C. impossible
   D. choice E. invasion

   2.____

3. _____ is usually defined as an excessively high rate of interest.

   A. Injustice B. Perjury C. Exorbitant
   D. Embezzlement E. Usury

   3.____

4. "I ask you, gentlemen of the jury, to find this man guilty since I have _____ the charges brought about him."

   A. documented B. questioned C. revised
   D. selected E. confused

   4.____

5. Although the critic was a close friend of the producer, he told him that he could not _____ his play.

   A. condemn B. prefer C. congratulate
   D. endorse E. revile

   5.____

6. Knowledge of human nature and motivation is an important _____ in all areas of endeavor.

   A. object B. incentive C. opportunity
   D. asset E. goal

   6.____

7. Numbered among the audience were kings, princes, dukes, and even a maharajah, all attempting to _____ another in the glitter of their habiliments and the number of their escorts.

   A. supersede B. outdo C. guide
   D. vanquish E. equal

   7.____

8. There seems to be a widespread feeling that peoples who are located below us in respect to latitude are _____ also in respect to intellect and ability.

   A. superior B. melodramatic C. inferior
   D. ulterior E. contemptible

   8.____

9. This should be considered a(n) _____ rather than the usual occurrence.   9.____

   A. coincidence   B. specialty   C. development
   D. outgrowth   E. mirage

10. Those who were considered states' rights adherents in the early part of our history, espoused the diminution of the powers of the national government because they had always been _____ of these powers.   10.____

    A. solicitous   B. advocates   C. apprehensive
    D. mindful   E. respectful

KEY (CORRECT ANSWERS)

1. E   6. D
2. A   7. B
3. E   8. C
4. A   9. A
5. D   10. C

TEST 6

DIRECTIONS: Each question in this section consists of a sentence in which one word is missing; a blank line indicates where the word has been removed from the sentence. Beneath each sentence are five words, *one* of which is the missing word. You are to select the letter of the missing word by deciding which one of the five words BEST fits in with the meaning of the sentence. *PRINT THE LETTER OF THE CORRECT ANSWER IN THE SPACE AT THE RIGHT.*

1. We can see in retrospect that the high hopes for lasting peace conceived at Versailles in 1919 were _____.

    A. ingenuous B. transient C. nostalgic
    D. ingenious E. specious

    1.____

2. One of the constructive effects of Nazism was the passage by the U.N. of a resolution to combat _____.

    A. armaments B. nationalism C. colonialism
    D. genocide E. geriatrics

    2.____

3. In our prisons, the role of _____ often gains for certain inmates a powerful position among their fellow prisoners.

    A. informer B. clerk C. warden D. trusty E. turnkey

    3.____

4. It is the _____ liar, experienced in the ways of the world, who finally trips upon some incongruous detail.

    A. consummate B. incorrigible C. congenital
    D. lagrant E. contemptible

    4.____

5. Anyone who is called a misogynist can hardly be expected to look upon women with _____ contemptuous eyes.

    A. more than B. nothing less than C. decidedly
    D. other than E. always

    5.____

6. Demagogues such as Hitler and Mussolini aroused the masses by appealing to their _____ rather than to their intellect.

    A. emotions B. reason C. nationalism
    D. conquests E. duty

    6.____

7. He was in great demand as an entertainer for his _____ abilities: he could sing, dance, tell a joke, or relate a story with equally great skill and facility.

    A. versatile B. logical C. culinary
    D. histrionic E. creative

    7.____

8. The wise politician is aware that, next to knowing when to seize an opportunity, it is also important to know when to _____ an advantage.

    A. develop B. seek C. revise
    D. proclaim E. forego

    8.____

9. Books on psychology inform us that the best way to break a bad habit is to _____ a new habit in its place.

   A. expel
   B. substitute
   C. conceal
   D. curtail
   E. supplant

10. The author who uses one word where another uses a whole paragraph, should be considered a _____ writer.

    A. successful
    B. grandiloquent
    C. experienced
    D. prolix
    E. succinct

KEY (CORRECT ANSWERS)

1. A
2. D
3. A
4. A
5. D
6. A
7. A
8. E
9. B
10. E

VERBAL ANALOGIES – 2 BLANKS
EXAMINATION SECTION
TEST 1

DIRECTIONS: Each question in this part consists of two capitalized words which have a certain relationship to each other, followed by four lettered pairs of words. Choose the letter of the pair of words which are related to each other in the SAME way as the words of the capitalized pair are related to each other. *PRINT THE LETTER OF THE CORRECT ANSWER IN THE SPACE AT THE RIGHT.*

1. BLUE : SKY ::
   A. new : path   B. tiny : mountain
   C. green : grass   D. glad : bear   1.____

2. EATING : DINING ROOM ::
   A. waiting : restaurant   B. cooking : kitchen
   C. sleeping : barn   D. running : bedroom   2.____

3. WASH : CLEAN ::
   A. iron : clothes   B. scrub : repair
   C. wipe : dry   D. rinse : dirty   3.____

4. HOT : COLD ::
   A. slow : easy   B. asleep : awake
   C. big : fat   D. funny : quick   4.____

5. LISTEN : RECORDS ::
   A. open : floor   B. jump : table
   C. meet : mile   D. watch : television   5.____

6. LEAD : PENCIL ::
   A. match : pipe   B. water : pail
   C. ink : pen   D. chalk : slate   6.____

7. DWARF : SMALL ::
   A. witch : stupid   B. clown : sad
   C. gnome : jolly   D. giant : tall   7.____

8. HOME RUN : BASEBALL ::
   A. round : wrestling   B. touchdown : football
   C. foul : basketball   D. drive : golf   8.____

9. CHICKEN : HATCHED ::
   A. baby : born   B. puppy : lost
   C. tree : planted   D. lawn : mowed   9.____

10. REMEMBER : FORGET ::
   A. find : lose   B. buy : own
   C. arrive : stay   D. borrow : rent   10.____

11. PIANO : KEY ::

    A. drum : bugle   B. guitar : string
    C. trumpet : band D. violin : case

12. KNAPSACK : HIKE ::

    A. suitcase : trip   B. sneaker : stroll
    C. canteen : journey D. bearer : safari

13. HEALTHY : SICK ::

    A. huge : large   B. rapid : sudden
    C. strong : weak   D. complete : empty

14. TENNIS : RACKET ::

    A. golf : club   B. chess : pawn
    C. checkers : board   D. boxing : ring

15. DORMITORY : SLEEPING ::

    A. theater : applauding B. classroom : learning
    C. truck : traveling   D. market : storing

16. SQUIRREL : NUTS ::

    A. termite : wood   B. grasshopper : sugar
    C. goat : milk   D. mouse : cheese

17. NEEDLE : SEW ::

    A. knife : carve   B. spoon : drink
    C. hammer : break   D. iron : steam

18. CORN : HUSK ::

    A. pea : pod   B. weed : flower
    C. spinach : leaf   D. plant : stem

19. MOTOR : GASOLINE ::

    A. bicycle : spoke   B. sailboat : wind
    C. engine : smoke   D. sled : ice

20. WALLET : MONEY ::

    A. notebook : paper   B. magazine : cover
    C. briefcase : leather   D. newspaper : print

21. FISH : CAT ::

    A. worm : bird   B. hoot : owl
    C. giraffe : beast   D. duck : goose

22. COFFEE : BEAN ::

    A. soda : flavor   B. cocoa : sugar
    C. tea : leaf   D. milk : cream

23. ABSENCE : ATTENDANCE ::

    A. emptiness : fullness
    B. peace : tranquility
    C. solemnity : gloom
    D. happiness : cheer

24. HAMMER : CARPENTER ::

    A. saw : janitor
    B. shovel : electrician
    C. wrench : plumber
    D. ladle : gardener

25. TIPTOE : STAMP ::

    A. practice : play
    B. sneak : attack
    C. whisper : shout
    D. hum : harmonize

26. WATER : LIQUID ::

    A. wood : hard
    B. cloth : pretty
    C. sand : yellow
    D. rock : solid

27. BRACELET : WRIST ::

    A. crutch : leg
    B. tooth : mouth
    C. lace : neck
    D. ring : finger

28. FLIGHT : AIRPLANE ::

    A. track : train
    B. garage : automobile
    C. voyage : ship
    D. destination : bus

29. ELEPHANT : TUSK ::

    A. rabbit : hare
    B. turtle : mud
    C. elk : antler
    D. alligator : swamp

30. DAIRY : MILK ::

    A. farm : egg
    B. bakery : bread
    C. factory : tool
    D. garden : tomato

31. FIRST : LAST ::

    A. today : tomorrow
    B. attempt : failure
    C. beginning : end
    D. length : width

32. TEMPERATURE : THERMOMETER ::

    A. year : calendar
    B. hour : second
    C. size : shape
    D. weight : scale

33. BOAT : CANAL ::

    A. yacht : anchor
    B. airplane : mechanic
    C. car : street
    D. bus : stop

34. FUDGE : CANDY ::

    A. rice : potato
    B. tuna : salmon
    C. fruit : vegetable
    D. lamb : meat

35. COLLAR : DOG ::
    A. fur : fox
    B. wing : sparrow
    C. bridle : horse
    D. cage : rabbit

    35._____

36. WOUND : HEAL ::
    A. bottle : break
    B. rip : mend
    C. wool : knit
    D. bump : hit

    36._____

37. CATERPILLAR : BUTTERFLY ::
    A. tadpole : frog
    B. ox : antelope
    C. pony : stallion
    D. mule : zebra

    37._____

38. ADMIRE : PRAISE ::
    A. dislike : criticize
    B. enjoy : memorize
    C. pretend : impress
    D. favor : persuade

    38._____

39. REFEREE : ROUND ::
    A. captain : team
    B. umpire : inning
    C. swimmer : pool
    D. player : match

    39._____

40. GROCER : VEGETABLES ::
    A. optometrist : eyes
    B. machinist : nails
    C. pharmacist : drugs
    D. typist : papers

    40._____

41. STOVE : HEATS ::
    A. refrigerator : cools
    B. sink : drains
    C. pot : boils
    D. toaster : burns

    41._____

42. GALE : WIND ::
    A. storm : weather
    B. downpour : rain
    C. humidity : moisture
    D. report : forecast

    42._____

43. KNEE : FOOT ::
    A. eye : ear
    B. fist : finger
    C. knuckle : nail
    D. elbow : hand

    43._____

44. BLUEPRINT : HOUSE ::
    A. script : theater
    B. map : globe
    C. skeleton : body
    D. pattern : dress

    44._____

45. TREE : FOREST ::
    A. gate : wall
    B. flower : bouquet
    C. house : street
    D. oil : drop

    45._____

46. GOOSE : FOWL ::
    A. crab : shellfish
    B. cow : calf
    C. eel : octopus
    D. worm : snake

    46._____

47. MUSIC : HEAR :: 47.____

    A. telephone : talk
    B. piano : touch
    C. quiz : solve
    D. picture : see

48. ZOO : MONKEY :: 48.____

    A. carnival : balloon
    B. aquarium : goldfish
    C. ranch : cowboy
    D. jungle : camel

49. PAINTER : BRUSH :: 49.____

    A. sculptor : chisel
    B. actor : script
    C. musician : baton
    D. architect : building

50. CHUM : FRIEND :: 50.____

    A. school : vacation
    B. hobby : interest
    C. game : enjoyment
    D. porch : house

KEY (CORRECT ANSWERS)

1. C	11. B	21. A	31. C	41. A
2. B	12. A	22. C	32. D	42. B
3. C	13. C	23. A	33. C	43. D
4. B	14. A	24. C	34. D	44. D
5. D	15. B	25. C	35. C	45. B
6. C	16. D	26. D	36. B	46. A
7. D	17. A	27. D	37. A	47. D
8. B	18. A	28. C	38. A	48. B
9. A	19. B	29. C	39. B	49. A
10. A	20. A	30. B	40. C	50. B

TEST 2

DIRECTIONS: Each question in this part consists of two capitalized words which have a certain relationship to each other, followed by four lettered pairs of words. Choose the letter of the pair of words which are related to each other in the SAME way as the words of the capitalized pair are related to each other. *PRINT THE LETTER OF THE CORRECT ANSWER IN THE SPACE AT THE RIGHT.*

1. LEAD : PENCIL ::

    A. match : pipe
    C. ink : pen
    B. water : pail
    D. chalk : slate

    1.____

2. DWARF : SMALL ::

    A. witch : stupid
    C. gnome : jolly
    B. clown : sad
    D. giant : tall

    2.____

3. BOOK : WRITE ::

    A. puzzle : add
    C. building : wreck
    B. picture : draw
    D. road : fix

    3.____

4. AIRPLANE : BIRD ::

    A. truck : eagle
    C. submarine : fish
    B. railroad : mule
    D. computer : owl

    4.____

5. KANGAROO : HOP ::

    A. cat : wander
    C. spider : fly
    B. snake : crawl
    D. crow : perch

    5.____

6. TENNIS : RACKET ::

    A. golf : club
    C. croquet : wicket
    B. chess : pawn
    D. boxing : ring

    6.____

7. DINNER : BANQUET ::

    A. car : limousine
    C. boat : sail
    B. bus : motorcycle
    D. train : track

    7.____

8. CHARIOT : HORSE ::

    A. den : bear
    C. hutch : rabbit
    B. wagon : cart
    D. automobile : engine

    8.____

9. HEALTHY : SICK ::

    A. huge : large
    C. strong : weak
    B. rapid : sudden
    D. complete : empty

    9.____

10. DINING ROOM : EAT ::

    A. kitchen : sit
    C. bedroom : sleep
    B. porch : read
    D. closet : hide

    10.____

11. FOUL : FAIR ::

    A. unlawful : legal
    C. complex : complicated
    B. good : better
    D. near : close

    11.____

12. DAGGER : SWORD ::

    A. pistol : rifle
    B. bow : arrow
    C. shell : bullet
    D. trigger : gun

    12.____

13. CAT : TIGER ::

    A. lizard : turtle
    B. dog : wolf
    C. bird : insect
    D. mare : cow

    13.____

14. DRAMATICS : THEATER ::

    A. acoustics : auditorium
    B. pediatrics : playground
    C. athletics : gymnasium
    D. economics : bank

    14.____

15. HAND BEATER : ELECTRIC MIXER ::

    A. broom : vacuum cleaner
    B. flashlight : light bulb
    C. sink : dishwasher
    D. wrench : vise

    15.____

16. COAST : OCEAN ::

    A. sand : beach
    B. grass : island
    C. tunnel : mountain
    D. bank : river

    16.____

17. PRESCRIPTION : MEDICINE ::

    A. recipe : cake
    B. food : meal
    C. pill : powder
    D. petition : name

    17.____

18. COCONUT : MILK ::

    A. grapefruit : juice
    B. peach : fuzz
    C. plum : jelly
    D. almond : nut

    18.____

19. CLASP : NECKLACE ::

    A. brooch : pin
    B. buckle : belt
    C. seam : garment
    D. thong : sandal

    19.____

20. MANUFACTURE : REFRIGERATORS ::

    A. publish : newspapers
    B. edit : manuscripts
    C. dye : fabrics
    D. repair : watches

    20.____

21. NUMB : FEELING ::

    A. blind : knowing
    B. deaf : hearing
    C. stiff : touching
    D. ill : tasting

    21.____

22. BASKETBALL : COURT ::

    A. target : revolver
    B. archery : range
    C. baseball : bleachers
    D. hockey : stick

    22.____

23. INITIATION : CLUB MEMBER ::

    A. introduction : letter
    B. imitation : mimic
    C. inauguration : president
    D. implication : speaker

    23.____

24. SAVE : WASTE ::
    - A. deny : disprove
    - B. hoard : withhold
    - C. acquire : inherit
    - D. accumulate : disperse

25. PRICK : PIN ::
    - A. break : dish
    - B. cut : knife
    - C. rip : scissors
    - D. punch : paper

26. VACATION : SCHOOL ::
    - A. finale : opera
    - B. recess : yard
    - C. margin : book
    - D. intermission : performance

27. LEGIBLE : WRITING ::
    - A. clear : thinking
    - B. swift : walking
    - C. soft : speaking
    - D. pretty : seeing

28. ORDER : DELIVER ::
    - A. prepare : destroy
    - B. wonder : think
    - C. ask : answer
    - D. find : lose

29. EXTORTIONIST : BLACKMAIL ::
    - A. arsonist : bail
    - B. kidnapper : crime
    - C. kleptomaniac : theft
    - D. bandit : reward

30. SNOWPLOW : SNOW ::
    - A. crane : rocks
    - B. tractor : farm
    - C. bulldozer : earth
    - D. tank : army

31. JAVELIN : THROW ::
    - A. stadium : sit
    - B. discus : weigh
    - C. rope : swing
    - D. hurdle : jump

32. TWINKLE : EYE ::
    - A. frown : wrinkle
    - B. grin : mouth
    - C. chuckle : laugh
    - D. anger : tears

33. KAYAK : CANOE ::
    - A. igloo : tepee
    - B. bow : arrow
    - C. child : papoose
    - D. blubber : wampum

34. BEDROCK : TOPSOIL ::
    - A. cellar : garage
    - B. house : porch
    - C. foundation : roof
    - D. fireplace : chimney

35. WETNESS : MONSOON ::
    - A. coldness : famine
    - B. mildness : season
    - C. windiness : rain
    - D. dryness : drought

36. QUARRY : GRANITE ::

    A. pond : brook
    B. mine : coal
    C. granary : wheat
    D. cliff : rock

37. TURPENTINE : PAINT ::

    A. polish : varnish
    B. soap : dirt
    C. cleaner : floor
    D. mop : rag

38. SPIKE : STAKE ::

    A. timber : lumber
    B. leather : hide
    C. nail : peg
    D. nut : bolt

39. BRIEFCASE : FILE CABINET ::

    A. letter : envelope
    B. wallet : vault
    C. satchel : pouch
    D. suitcase : luggage

40. AMATEUR : PROFESSIONAL ::

    A. teacher : professor
    B. writer : editor
    C. beginner : veteran
    D. prompter : understudy

41. MIRAGE : ILLUSION ::

    A. object : reality
    B. happiness : tragedy
    C. plan : obstacle
    D. pain : relief

42. HUSK : CORN ::

    A. seed : flower
    B. leaf : stem
    C. cob : stalk
    D. pod : pea

43. BUTTON : HOLE ::

    A. zipper : lining
    B. snap : fastener
    C. hook : eye
    D. stitch : hem

44. ATTIC : HOUSE ::

    A. peak : mountain
    B. bush : tree
    C. top : bottom
    D. hill : slope

45. STOMACH : DIGESTION ::

    A. blood : circulation
    B. gland : sensation
    C. skeleton : posture
    D. lung : respiration

46. SHIELD : PROTECTION ::

    A. armor : insulation
    B. disguise : deception
    C. flag : attention
    D. war : duration

47. FLICKER : FLAME ::

    A. nod : head
    B. break : wave
    C. quench : fire
    D. quaver : voice

48. BURLAP : SILK ::

    A. material : velvet
    B. needle : thread
    C. pottery : china
    D. plate : bowl

49. SKYSCRAPER : URBAN ::

    A. highway : metropolitan
    B. apartment : local
    C. garage : surburban
    D. silo : rural

50. CINNAMON : SPICE ::

    A. mustard : condiment
    B. sauce : herb
    C. liqueur : appetizer
    D. icing : dessert

KEY (CORRECT ANSWERS)

1. C	11. A	21. B	31. D	41. A
2. D	12. A	22. B	32. B	42. D
3. B	13. B	23. C	33. C	43. C
4. C	14. C	24. D	34. C	44. A
5. B	15. A	25. B	35. D	45. D
6. A	16. A	26. D	36. B	46. B
7. A	17. A	27. A	37. B	47. B
8. D	18. A	28. A	38. C	48. C
9. C	19. A	29. C	39. B	49. D
10. C	20. A	30. C	40. C	50. A

TEST 3

DIRECTIONS: Each question in this part consists of two capitalized words which have a certain relationship to each other, followed by four lettered pairs of words. Choose the letter of the pair of words which are related to each other in the SAME way as the words of the capitalized pair are related to each other. *PRINT THE LETTER OF THE CORRECT ANSWER IN THE SPACE AT THE RIGHT.*

1. COMMA : PERIOD ::　　　　　　　　　　　　　　　　　　　　　　　　　　1.____
   A. begin : cease　　　　　　　　　B. cut : sever
   C. delay : hinder　　　　　　　　　D. pause : stop

2. IRON : RUST ::　　　　　　　　　　　　　　　　　　　　　　　　　　　　2.____
   A. steel : bend　　　　　　　　　　B. silver : tarnish
   C. wood : crumble　　　　　　　　　D. gold : melt

3. RACETRACK : BET ::　　　　　　　　　　　　　　　　　　　　　　　　　　3.____
   A. opera : sing　　　　　　　　　　B. circus : perform
   C. auction : bid　　　　　　　　　　D. bazaar : display

4. COPYRIGHT : PUBLISHED ::　　　　　　　　　　　　　　　　　　　　　　　4.____
   A. requirement : completed　　　　B. patent : manufactured
   C. plaque : remembered　　　　　　D. deed : purchased

5. CANARY : CAGE ::　　　　　　　　　　　　　　　　　　　　　　　　　　　5.____
   A. bear : cave　　　　　　　　　　　B. squirrel : tree
   C. horse : racecourse　　　　　　　D. goldfish : aquarium

6. PURITY : TAINTED ::　　　　　　　　　　　　　　　　　　　　　　　　　6.____
   A. hardiness : healthy　　　　　　B. tastiness : aged
   C. freshness : stale　　　　　　　D. coldness : icy

7. GERM : DISINFECT ::　　　　　　　　　　　　　　　　　　　　　　　　　7.____
   A. insect : exterminate　　　　　　B. fat : saturate
   C. vapor : fumigate　　　　　　　　D. root : cultivate

8. RINK : SKATE ::　　　　　　　　　　　　　　　　　　　　　　　　　　　8.____
   A. stadium : sit　　　　　　　　　　B. arena : cheer
   C. pool : swim　　　　　　　　　　　D. snow : ski

9. SKIRMISH : BATTLE ::　　　　　　　　　　　　　　　　　　　　　　　　　9.____
   A. tiff : fight　　　　　　　　　　　B. soldier : company
   C. advance : retreat　　　　　　　　D. camp : fort

10. IDENTICAL : DIFFERENCES ::　　　　　　　　　　　　　　　　　　　　　10.____
    A. dynamic : exceptions　　　　　　B. symmetrical : details
    C. perfect : flaws　　　　　　　　　D. intact : parts

11. DOCTOR : SURGEON ::

    A. artist : sculptor
    B. lawyer : official
    C. actor : director
    D. clerk : supervisor

12. FORGE : SIGNATURE ::

    A. repeat : order
    B. sketch : illustration
    C. gamble : dice
    D. counterfeit : money

13. ALMOND : NUT ::

    A. honey : flower
    B. leaf : branch
    C. apricot : fruit
    D. corn : kernel

14. FOURSOME : GOLF ::

    A. team : playing
    B. band : marching
    C. singles : serving
    D. quartet : singing

15. BUCK : DOE ::

    A. panther : cub
    B. calf : bull
    C. ram : ewe
    D. raven : crow

16. PROTECT : RESCUE ::

    A. preserve : waste
    B. procure : receive
    C. prevent : cure
    D. promote : deter

17. IRONING : WRINKLES ::

    A. dusting : mops
    B. cleaning : stains
    C. sewing : seams
    D. cooking : odors

18. BEAUTICIAN : HAIR ::

    A. barber : chin
    B. speaker : tongue
    C. manicurist : nails
    D. chiropodist : toes

19. TICK : CLOCK ::

    A. buzzer : doorbell
    B. ring : telephone
    C. tap : step
    D. pitch : voice

20. IMPOUND : DOG ::

    A. levy : revenue
    B. license : hunter
    C. imprison : person
    D. inspect : baggage

21. HAZY : SIGHT ::

    A. salty : taste
    B. pungent : smell
    C. shiny : touch
    D. muffled : sound

22. STUDENT : TUITION ::

    A. minister : collection
    B. employee : taxation
    C. traveler : trip
    D. tenant : rent

23. UMPIRE : BASEBALL ::
    A. center : basketball
    B. jockey : racing
    C. referee : boxing
    D. goalie : soccer

24. TOOL : HAMMER ::
    A. ornament : ribbon
    B. metal : structure
    C. needle : scissors
    D. velvet : sheen

25. IMPORTED : DOMESTIC ::
    A. alien : native
    B. senator : enactment
    C. musician : performer
    D. deacon : congregation

26. THIEF : STEALS ::
    A. perjurer : lies
    B. pirate : sails
    C. murderer : hides
    D. saboteur : kidnaps

27. COW : BOVINE ::
    A. kennel : canine
    B. trout : aquatic
    C. cat : feline
    D. bird : aerial

28. THIMBLE : FINGER ::
    A. ankles : shins
    B. goggles : eyes
    C. bracelet : wrist
    D. belt : waist

29. BASE : PYRAMID ::
    A. angle : corner
    B. floor : room
    C. height : house
    D. pot : flower

30. THEORY : APPLICATION ::
    A. thought : action
    B. experiment : apparatus
    C. research : finding
    D. machine : production

31. ENCYCLOPEDIA : INFORMATION ::
    A. verse : reference
    B. index : definition
    C. manual : instruction
    D. textbook : activity

32. CREDIBLE : CERTAIN ::
    A. possible : actual
    B. indefinite : undecided
    C. careless : thoughtful
    D. factual : real

33. SOPORIFIC : SLEEPINESS ::
    A. stimulant : alertness
    B. tranquilizer : nervousness
    C. medicine : disease
    D. aspirin : headache

34. APOLOGIZE : SORRY ::
    A. complain : discontent
    B. rationalize : emotional
    C. submit : recalcitrant
    D. antagonize : placid

35. INVITATION : GUEST ::
    A. mortgage : owner
    B. subpoena : witness
    C. certificate : notary
    D. diploma : graduate

36. RUSHED : TIME ::
    A. frantic : motion
    B. busy : idea
    C. cramped : space
    D. nimble : position

37. WARDEN : PRISON ::
    A. porter : depot
    B. janitor : office
    C. painter : gallery
    D. curator : museum

38. ESSAY : WORD ::
    A. code : letter
    B. sonata : note
    C. graph : number
    D. algebra : line

39. MIND : CLEVER ::
    A. soul : unseen
    B. body : agile
    C. form : slender
    D. notion : fanciful

40. BLIGHT : PLANTS ::
    A. famine : crops
    B. drought : land
    C. plague : people
    D. fire : timber

41. VOCALIST : SONGS ::
    A. musician : compositions
    B. engineer : highways
    C. athlete : teams
    D. orator : speeches

42. TRIBUTE : PRAISE ::
    A. criticism : admiration
    B. denouncement : censure
    C. drama : action
    D. poetry : prose

43. FOWL : TURKEY ::
    A. carnivore : beef
    B. legume : bean
    C. carrot : stalk
    D. head : lettuce

44. PRIDE : CONCEIT ::
    A. humility : vanity
    B. weakness : strength
    C. prejudice : dislike
    D. caution : cowardice

45. EQUAL : EXCEED ::
    A. colleague : friend
    B. runner-up : winner
    C. peer : superior
    D. helper : partner

46. NATURALIZATION : CITIZENSHIP ::
    A. conversion : religion
    B. change : chameleon
    C. representation : statehood
    D. vote : franchise

47. PIOUS : SANCTIMONIOUS ::

    A. dignified : pompous
    B. intelligent : witty
    C. skillful : nimble
    D. curious : uninformed

48. INSERT : DELETE ::

    A. approve : edit
    B. alter : revise
    C. whiten : darken
    D. lengthen : shorten

49. SHAWL : COAT ::

    A. kerchief : hat
    B. hood : cape
    C. scarf : glove
    D. boot : shoe

50. INFRACTION : LAW ::

    A. ignorance : rule
    B. faith : belief
    C. learning : education
    D. crudity : propriety

KEY (CORRECT ANSWERS)

1. D	11. A	21. D	31. C	41. A
2. B	12. D	22. D	32. A	42. B
3. C	13. C	23. C	33. A	43. B
4. D	14. D	24. A	34. A	44. D
5. D	15. C	25. A	35. D	45. C
6. C	16. C	26. A	36. C	46. A
7. A	17. B	27. C	37. D	47. A
8. C	18. C	28. B	38. B	48. D
9. A	19. B	29. B	39. B	49. B
10. C	20. C	30. A	40. A	50. A

VERBAL ANALOGIES
EXAMINATION SECTION
TEST 1

DIRECTIONS: Each question consists of two capitalized words which have a certain relationship to each other, followed by five lettered pairs of words in small letters. Choose the letter of the pair of words which are related to each other in the SAME way as the words of the capitalized pair are related to each other. *PRINT THE LETTER OF THE CORRECT ANSWER IN THE SPACE AT THE RIGHT.*

1. DISEASE : IMMUNITY :: _____ : _____ 1.____
   A. crime : pardon   B. custom : practice   C. debt : bankruptcy
   D. tax : exemption   E. travel : deduction

2. RESPONSIBILITY : RELEASE :: _____ : _____ 2.____
   A. duty : refrain   B. promise : renege   C. debt : honor
   D. blame : vindicate   E. position : retract

3. PENDULUM : SWING :: _____ : _____ 3.____
   A. pulley : ladder   B. hand : clock   C. lever : crowbar
   D. balance : seesaw   E. weight : fulcrum

4. NADIR : ZENITH :: _____ : _____ 4.____
   A. depression : recovery   B. perigee : apogamy
   C. earth : sky   D. appanage : station
   E. threshold : lintel

5. ROB : CONFISCATE :: _____ : _____ 5.____
   A. punish : revenge   B. walk : trespass   C. insult : offend
   D. murder : execute   E. take : accept

6. WORKER : UNEMPLOYED :: _____ : _____ 6.____
   A. crop : barren   B. property : useless
   C. purchase : unnecessary   D. visitor : unwelcome
   E. field : fallow

7. PROFUSION : AUSTERITY :: _____ : _____ 7.____
   A. capitalism : socialism   B. erudition : reprise
   C. logic : irrationality   D. affluence : frugality
   E. effluence : confluence

8. REPERTOIRE : OPERA :: _____ : _____ 8.____
   A. suits : closet   B. team : baseball   C. melody : harmony
   D. wardrobe : costume   E. chest : drawers

9. DISDAIN : AFFRONT :: _____ : _____
   A. perjury : boos
   B. pleasure : pain
   C. approval : applause
   D. age : wrinkle
   E. grimace : awry

10. SALES : ADVERTISING :: _____ : _____
    A. votes : campaigning
    B. savings : banking
    C. liquor : drinking
    D. troops : leading
    E. weakness : strength

11. ATTACK : MURDER :: _____ : _____
    A. filial : fraternal
    B. mind : body
    C. paroxysm : parricide
    D. sudden : poison
    E. diseased : dead

12. BALTIC : INDIAN :: _____ : _____
    A. Mediterranean : Pacific
    B. Atlantic : Caribbean
    C. Arctic : Gulf of Mexico
    D. Black Sea : Persian Gulf
    E. Antarctic : Andaman Sea

13. PROFESSION : STRUGGLE :: _____ : _____
    A. strong : weak
    B. métier : melee
    C. mixed : confusion
    D. vocation : trade
    E. expert : novice

14. ALLOYS : ATMOSPHERE :: _____ : _____
    A. weight : measure
    B. metallurgy : meteorology
    C. technology : science
    D. archaic : present

15. GRAM : KILOGRAM :: _____ : _____
    A. millimeter : centimeter
    B. dekameter : decimeter
    C. mile : kilometer
    D. micron : microbe
    E. Centigrade : Fahrenheit

16. PRESIDENT : FRANCE :: _____ : _____
    A. Queen Elizabeth : England
    B. king : Belgium
    C. president : United States
    D. governor : state
    E. king : Italy

17. HAND : DIAL :: _____ : _____
    A. time : number
    B. light : lamp
    C. ticking : talking
    D. clock : radio
    E. time : space

18. ANNEX : BUILDING :: _____ : _____
    A. pin : clasp
    B. stone : setting
    C. cell : prison
    D. branch : tree
    E. island : mainland

19. FLOOR : PARQUET :: _____ : _____
    A. elevator : escalator
    B. functional : ornamental
    C. filigree : scroll
    D. wreath : nosegay
    E. head : hair

3 (#1)

20. DEVIL : DRUGGIST :: _____ : _____   20._____
    A. demon : farmer   B. demonology : pharmacology
    C. medieval : primitive   D. dispensed : compounded
    E. Faustian : Freudian

21. ELECTRICITY : GAS :: _____ : _____   21._____
    A. lighter : match   B. current : flow   C. fire : flame
    D. conductor : ignition   E. train : automobile

22. - : HYPHEN :: _____ : _____   22._____
    A. x : division   B. $: pound   C. symbol : word
    D. y : geometry   E. & : sum

23. WILD : DOMESTICATED :: _____ : _____   23._____
    A. jungle : forest   B. atavistic : masochistic
    C. cave : dwelling   D. animal : man
    E. primitive : civilized

24. INEPT : TACTLESS :: _____ : _____   24._____
    A. right : left   B. evil : sinful   C. clever : stupid
    D. depraved : foolish   E. maladroit : gauche

25. INTERVENE : INTERCEDE :: _____ : _____   25._____
    A. interfere : impute   B. interpose : intrude   C. arbitrate : argue
    D. meditate : mediate   E. space : species

KEY (CORRECT ANSWERS)

1. D
2. D
3. C
4. E
5. D

6. E
7. D
8. D
9. C
10. A

11. C
12. A
13. B
14. B
15. A

16. C
17. D
18. D
19. B
20. B

21. B
22. C
23. E
24. E
25. B

TEST 2

DIRECTIONS: Each question consists of two capitalized words which have a certain relationship to each other, followed by five lettered pairs of words in small letters. Choose the letter of the pair of words which are related to each other in the SAME way as the words of the capitalized pair are related to each other. *PRINT THE LETTER OF THE CORRECT ANSWER IN THE SPACE AT THE RIGHT.*

1. PITHY : BOMBASTIC :: _____ : _____
   A. verbose : taciturn   B. garrulous : pompous
   C. meagre : replete   D. laconic : grandiloquent
   E. concise : precise

2. MANAGER : TEAM :: _____ : _____
   A. President : Congress   B. Speaker : Senate
   C. captain : crew   D. minister : hierarchy
   E. principal : P.T.A.

3. STEEPLE : LEDGE :: _____ : _____
   A. citadel : tower   B. spire : dungeon   C. warp : woof
   D. peak : summit   E. cone : roof

4. CREDULOUS : UNCTUOUS :: _____ : _____
   A. ingenious : artful   B. ingenuous : urbane
   C. naïve : provincial   D. benign : benignant
   E. cantankerous : peevish

5. PHILIPPIC : ABUSE :: _____ : _____
   A. eulogy : mirth   B. tirade : tears   C. sycophancy : music
   D. encomium : praise   E. intrepidity : fear

6. CUMULATIVE : ACCRETIVE :: _____ : _____
   A. indigenous : spontaneous   B. reticence : verbosity
   C. philately : numismatics   D. indigence : poverty
   E. culvert : bridge

7. UNCONSTRAINED : IMPROVISED :: _____ : _____
   A. unrehearsed : prepared   B. simultaneous : pithy
   C. premeditated : unpremeditated   D. extemporaneous : contemporaneous
   E. spontaneous : impromptu

8. INORDINACY : EXCESSIVE :: _____ : _____
   A. applause : approval   B. anomaly : irregular
   C. remuneration : payable   D. provocation : irritate
   E. emulation : insidious

9. PLEBEIAN : PATRICIAN :: _____ : _____
   A. Democrat : Republican
   B. Communist : Conservative
   C. serf : fief
   D. vassal : lord
   E. common man : elite

10. FLEETING : EPHEMERAL :: _____ : _____
    A. permanent : temporary
    B. casual : persistent
    C. transient : evanescent
    D. temporary : permanent
    E. passing : perceptible

11. INSTRUMENTALIST : ORGANIST :: _____ : _____
    A. harmonist : contrapuntist
    B. quartet : counterpoint
    C. lute : lutenist
    D. singer : composition
    E. cello : violoncello

12. ADULTERATE : COMPOUND :: _____ : _____
    A. fusión : blend
    B. commingle : miscellany
    C. interpretation : commingling
    D. interpolate : amalgamate
    E. mix : potpourri

13. QUIESCENCE : INDOLENCE :: _____ : _____
    A. lurk : abeyance
    B. concealed : potential
    C. latency : dormancy
    D. escape : observation
    E. suppress : inertia

14. BROGUE : JARGONIST :: _____ : _____
    A. patois : neologist
    B. empathy : psychiatrist
    C. dialect : Anglicism
    D. country : patriot
    E. gazette : journalist

15. DENIAL : DISCLAIMER :: _____ : _____
    A. veto : ignore
    B. contradiction : convention
    C. cancel : canker
    D. disavowal : negation
    E. gainsay : contradict

16. FATE : PREDESTINATION :: _____ : _____
    A. doom : destiny
    B. appointed : office
    C. elect : fated
    D. exigency : inevitability
    E. lot : choice

17. LETHARGY : EXHAUSTION :: _____ : _____
    A. laziness : weariness
    B. continence : ennui
    C. enfeebled : haggard
    D. exertion : tiredness
    E. lassitude : fatigue

18. QUALM : IRRESOLUTION :: _____ : _____
    A. fear : diffidence
    B. fright : stampede
    C. awe : trust
    D. sanguine : apprehensive
    E. nightmare : alarm

3 (#2)

19. WAR : SURRENDER :: _____ : _____
    A. victor : accede B. grant : scholarship C. election : concede
    D. state : cede E. prison : confess

    19._____

20. BALD EAGLE : GROUSE :: _____ : _____
    A. termite : cockroach B. chanticleer : rooster C. falcon : pheasant
    D. peacock : hen E. vulture : hawk

    20._____

21. ORANGUTAN : BRONCHO :: _____ : _____
    A. antelope : trotter
    B. Wales : United States
    C. caribou : marmoset
    D. ewe : ram
    E. steeplechaser : pacer

    21._____

22. UNITED STATES : FRANCE :: _____ : _____
    A. official : citizen
    B. policeman : gendarme
    C. officer : attendant
    D. New York : Louisiana
    E. west : east

    22._____

23. SEOUL : SOUTH KOREA :: _____ : _____
    A. Estopil : Portugal B. Pnom Penh : Laos C. Barcelona : Spain
    C. London : England E. Venezuela : Caracas

    23._____

24. PERSECUTION : PARANOIA :: _____ : _____
    A. altruism : megalomania
    B. neurosis : psychosis
    C. dichotomy : schizophrenia
    D. extraversion : claustrophobia
    E. disease : symptom

    24._____

25. ONE : TWO :: _____ : _____
    A. century : millennium
    B. planet : astronomy
    C. year : twenty
    D. month : year
    E. decade : score

    25._____

KEY (CORRECT ANSWERS)

1. D
2. C
3. C
4. B
5. D

6. D
7. E
8. B
9. E
10. C

11. A
12. D
13. C
14. A
15. D

16. A
17. E
18. A
19. C
20. C

21. A
22. B
23. D
24. C
25. E

TEST 3

DIRECTIONS: Each question consists of two capitalized words which have a certain relationship to each other, followed by five lettered pairs of words in small letters. Choose the letter of the pair of words which are related to each other in the SAME way as the words of the capitalized pair are related to each other. *PRINT THE LETTER OF THE CORRECT ANSWER IN THE SPACE AT THE RIGHT.*

1. CHAFFER : BARGAIN :: _____ : _____   1.____
   A. scarify : cleanse   B. hector : befriend
   C. propitiate : placate   D. improvise : intercalate
   E. decollate : decode

2. SPANIEL : FAWNING PERSON :: _____ : _____   2.____
   A. cameo : miniature   B. nonage : minority   C. pediment : obstacle
   D. flacon : flag   E. marasca : wine

3. SEMINAL : ORIGINATIVE :: _____ : _____   3.____
   A. sullied : inflamed   B. beleaguered : besieged
   C. viable : moribund   D. amorphous : remanent
   E. quintan : fourth

4. SLAKE : ALLAY :: _____ : _____   4.____
   A. comport : frolic   B. beset : assail   C. parry : join
   D. revet : review   E. remonstrate : concur

5. SALAAM : OBEISANCE :: _____ : _____   5.____
   A. jape : hiatus   B. ethos : fundamental spirit of a culture
   C. gravamen : greeting   D. chanticleer : fox
   E. ablation : inhalation

6. SLATTERNLY : SLOVENLY :: _____ : _____   6.____
   A. complaisant : priggish   B. myopic : farsighted
   C. awry : convex   D. oblate : flattened at the poles
   E. slavish : sleazy

7. PREEN : SLEEK :: _____ : _____   7.____
   A. extrapolate : disengage   B. discountenance : disconcert
   C. bandy : banter   D. cense : ascribe
   E. cite : proscribe

8. SATRAP : EXECUTE :: _____ : _____   8.____
   A. rigmarole : prolix talk   B. apostasy : denunciation
   C. apogee : perigee   D. allotrophy : allusion
   E. chaldron : chalice

2 (#3)

9. INCHOATE : NASCENT :: _____ : _____   9._____
   A. extirpative : invective   B. contumacious : headstrong
   C. disinterested : prejudiced   D. veracious : mendacious
   E. abandoned : manumitted

10. RAIL : REVILE :: _____ : _____   10._____
    A. abjure : appeal to   B. vouchsafe : contemplate
    C. execrate : curse   D. exorcise : criticize
    E. ablactate : abominate

11. ANTONYM : OPPOSITE :: _____ : _____   11._____
    A. antonym : unlike   B. metaphor : poetry
    C. triangle : pyramid   D. synonym : sme
    E. metonymy : versification

12. READER : PUNCTUATION :: _____ : _____   12._____
    A. telegraph operator : Morse   B. vocabulary : alphabet
    C. English : pronunciation   D. bicyclist : roadblock
    E. motorist : road sign

13. OCEAN : ROAD :: _____ : _____   13._____
    A. ship : hurricane   B. canal : road   C. storm : accident
    D. buoy : detour   E. warning : signal

14. MATTER : ESSENCE :: _____ : _____   14._____
    A. play : outcome   B. matter : particle   C. molecule : atom
    D. paragraph : gist   E. epitome : paraphrase

15. PENURIOUS : SLUM :: _____ : _____   15._____
    A. captive : jail   B. parched : desert   C. withered : plant
    D. inundated : flood   E. glum : outlook

16. DEMEANOR : CHARACTER :: _____ : _____   16._____
    A. personality : qualities   B. aspect : appearance
    C. vestibule : apartment   D. facade : building
    E. front : affront

17. HAIR : TRIM :: _____ : _____   17._____
    A. beard : shave   B. lawn : mow   C. wool : shear
    D. shrub : prune   E. scissors : cut

18. WORK : PUTTER :: _____ : _____   18._____
    A. bum : thief   B. late : laggard   C. regress : ingress
    D. diligent : tardy   E. wait : loiter

19. EXILE : SANCTUARY :: _____ : _____   19._____
    A. child : bed   B. refugee : haven   C. berth : stowaway
    D. fish : bowl   E. prisoner : dungeon

20. CAR : HORN :: _____ : _____
    A. air raid : siren   B. swimmer : bell buoy   C. singer : tune
    D. train : whistle   E. ship : anchor

21. SETTING : DIAMOND :: _____ : _____
    A. sash : window   B. frame : picture   C. shell : egg
    D. painting : canvas   E. border : exile

22. AFFECTION : PASSION :: _____ : _____
    A. storm : sea   B. contraction : dilation
    C. atmospheric pressure : clear day D. breeze : gale
    E. wind : gale

23. TEAR : CUT :: _____ : _____
    A. wrinkle : fold   B. paper : refuse   C. wrinkle : smooth
    D. steal : lose   E. sprinkle : rub

24. FIGHTER : BELL :: _____ : _____
    A. butterfly hunter : net   B. fencer : sword
    C. writer : pen   D. dog : whistle
    E. sprinter : gun

25. PLANT : FUNGUS :: _____ : _____
    A. transient : permanent   B. mate : captain
    C. sailor : pirate   D. police : thief
    E. wolf : prey

KEY (CORRECT ANSWERS)

1.	C	11.	D
2.	B	12.	E
3.	B	13.	D
4.	B	14.	D
5.	B	15.	B
6.	D	16.	D
7.	B	17.	D
8.	A	18.	E
9.	B	19.	B
10.	C	20.	D

21.	B
22.	E
23.	A
24.	E
25.	C

TEST 4

DIRECTIONS: Each question consists of two capitalized words which have a certain relationship to each other, followed by five lettered pairs of words in small letters. Choose the letter of the pair of words which are related to each other in the SAME way as the words of the capitalized pair are related to each other. *PRINT THE LETTER OF THE CORRECT ANSWER IN THE SPACE AT THE RIGHT.*

1. EVENING : MORNING :: _____ : _____
   A. coming : going
   B. ten : five
   C. sunset : sunrise
   D. spring : autumn
   E. despair : hope

2. RUNG : RING :: _____ : _____
   A. arisen : arise
   B. drunk : drink
   C. stroke : strike
   D. sang : sing
   E. clang : cling

3. ENTHUSIASTIC : APPROVING :: _____ : _____
   A. disliking : liking
   B. pink : red
   C. frigid : cool
   D. bitter : sour
   E. apathetic : disapproving

4. MOLECULE : ATOM :: _____ : _____
   A. kennel : dog
   B. shelf : book
   C. sea : fish
   D. regiment : soldier
   E. star : galaxy

5. ACT : PLAY :: _____ : _____
   A. notes : staff
   B. harmony : counterpoint
   C. melody : harmony
   D. key : piano
   E. movement : symphony

6. APIARY : BEES :: _____ : _____
   A. dog : kennel
   B. fish : aquarium
   C. mortuary : people
   D. corral : cattle
   E. breviary : priest

7. STRANDS : ROPE :: _____ : _____
   A. sugar : cane
   B. warp : woof
   C. links : chain
   D. train : cars
   E. rivers : ocean

8. BODY : SKIN :: _____ : _____
   A. window : door
   B. ink : crayon
   C. book : cover
   D. write : compose
   E. spelling : grammar

9. PENCIL : LEAD :: _____ : _____
   A. lighter : fluid
   B. keys : typewriter
   C. cup : coffee
   D. book : page
   E. razor : blade

10. AIRPLANE : LOCOMOTION :: _____ : _____
    A. statement : contention   B. canoe : paddle
    C. hero : worship   D. spectacles : vision
    E. hay : horse

11. STREAM : RIVER :: _____ : _____
    A. land : water   B. village : suburb   C. cape : continent
    D. sea : ocean   E. city : country

12. RECTANGLE : SQUARE :: _____ : _____
    A. line : perimeter   B. triangle : square   C. square : diamond
    D. circle : square   E. oval : circle

13. EMOLUMENT : INCENTIVE :: _____ : _____
    A. deed : crime   B. play : plot   C. criminal : reward
    D. dance : movement   E. reward : capture

14. WOLF : PROWL :: _____ : _____
    A. rat : gnaw   B. monkey : mimic   C. reader : browse
    D. trooper : lurk   E. gang : highjack

15. FOND : INFATUATION :: _____ : _____
    A. affectionate : adumbration
    C. eager : sentimentality
    E. enthusiastic : fervor
    B. calm : listless
    D. glib : fluency

16. CONCORD : DISCORD :: _____ : _____
    A. alliance : organization
    C. conciliation : revolution
    E. pact : feud
    B. treaty : covenant
    D. entreaty : parity

17. EXTENUATE : CRIME :: _____ : _____
    A. condone : error   B. placate : pardon   C. expiate : sin
    D. moderate : tone   E. reprisal : retaliation

18. APPENDIX : PREFACE :: _____ : _____
    A. glossary : index
    C. progeny : proletariat
    E. epilogue : prologue
    B. preface : table of contents
    D. footnote : emendation

19. SUBSEQUENT : COINCIDENTAL :: _____ : _____
    A. posthumous : following
    C. consecutive : ensuing
    E. prolonged : before
    B. now : there
    D. posterior : simultaneous

20. MUNDANE : SPIRITUAL :: _____ : _____
    A. scientist : missionary
    C. municipal : ecclesiastical
    E. student : teacher
    B. secular : altruistic
    D. pecuniary : musical

21. UNSCRUPULOUS : QUALMS :: _____ : _____ 21.____
    A. remorseless : compassion   B. intrepid : rashness
    C. opportunist : opportunity   D. querulous : lamentation
    E. impenitent : sin

22. SOPHISTRY : LOGIC :: _____ : _____ 22.____
    A. discretion : improvidence   B. spirit : spiritualism
    C. reason : rationalization   D. feeling : intuition
    E. wisdom : sophistication

23. TRESPASSER : BARK :: _____ : _____ 23.____
    A. snake : hiss   B. burglar : alarm   C. crossing : bell
    D. air raid : siren E. ship : buoy

24. RESEARCH : FELLOWSHIP :: _____ : _____ 24.____
    A. honor : medal   B. merit : scholarship C. student : bonus
    D. matrimony : dowry E. study : grant

25. IMPEND : DEMISE :: _____ : _____ 25.____
    A. loom : disaster   B. question : puzzle   C. imminent : eminent
    D. howl : storm   E. hurt : penalty

KEY (CORRECT ANSWERS)

1.	C	11.	D
2.	B	12.	E
3.	D	13.	E
4.	E	14.	E
5.	E	15.	E
6.	D	16.	E
7.	C	17.	A
8.	C	18.	E
9.	E	19.	D
10.	D	20.	B

21. A
22. D
23. B
24. E
25. A

TEST 5

DIRECTIONS: Each question consists of two capitalized words which have a certain relationship to each other, followed by five lettered pairs of words in small letters. Choose the letter of the pair of words which are related to each other in the SAME way as the words of the capitalized pair are related to each other. *PRINT THE LETTER OF THE CORRECT ANSWER IN THE SPACE AT THE RIGHT.*

1. DEATH : DEMISE :: _____ : _____   1._____
   A. frightful : horrid   B. resistance : invasion
   C. asylum : insane   D. life : breath
   E. might : right

2. DRAGON : DINOSAUR :: _____ : _____   2._____
   A. descendant : ancestor   B. medieval : prehistoric
   C. fabulous : real   D. creditable : veritable
   E. amphibian : reptile

3. SHIP : NAVIGATION :: _____ : _____   3._____
   A. promoter : event   B. victory : leader
   C. conduct : conscience   D. state : army
   E. nation : patriotism

4. GUFFAW : LAUGH :: _____ : _____   4._____
   A. lament : cry   B. wail : whimper   C. face : mouth
   D. chuckle : snicker   E. smirk : simper

5. ANARCHY : CHAOS :: _____ : _____   5._____
   A. government : order   B. beast : beauty   C. government : law
   D. rule : order   E. totalitarian : mob

6. INFINITE : FINITE :: _____ : _____   6._____
   A. second : minute   B. hour : minute   C. era : decade
   D. month : day   E. immortality : mortality

7. WATER : BOAT :: _____ : _____   7._____
   A. locomotive : steam   B. wagon : horse   C. air : dirigible
   D. lion : tiger   E. gasoline : taxi

8. INAUGURATION : PRESIDENT :: _____ : _____   8._____
   A. promulgation : list   B. matriculation : student
   C. election : candidate   D. promotion : officer
   E. ordination : priest

9. OMNIPOTENT : VASSAL :: _____ : _____   9._____
   A. soldier : civilian   B. policeman : prisoner
   C. master : slave   D. captain : tar
   E. native : alien

10. SAME : SYNONYM :: _____ : _____   10.____
    A. bell : bellows   B. false : pseudonym   C. same : homonym
    D. botanist : biologist   E. opposite : antonym

KEY (CORRECT ANSWERS)

1.	A	6.	E
2.	C	7.	C
3.	C	8.	E
4.	B	9.	C
5.	A	10.	E

DENTAL FUNDAMENTALS

CONTENTS

	Page
1. ANATOMY OF THE HEAD AND NECK	1
2. DENTAL ANATOMY	6
3. DENTAL HISTOLOGY	13

DENTAL FUNDAMENTALS

ANATOMY OF THE HEAD AND NECK

   Cranial Bones
   Facial Bones

      Landmarks of the Maxillae
      Landmarks of the Mandible

   Muscles of Mastication
   Structures of the Respiratory System

DENTAL ANATOMY

   Functions of the Teeth
   Location of the Teeth
   Identification of the Teeth
   Surfaces of the Teeth
   Anatomical Landmarks
   Occlusal Relationships

DENTAL HISTOLOGY

   Tissues of the Teeth

      Enamel
      Dentin
      Cementum
      Pulp

   Tissues of the Periodontium

      Alveolar Process
      Periodontal Ligament
      Gingiva

A knowledge of dental fundamentals is essential to the dental assistant. You will use this knowledge every day, when you complete dental records and other related forms, and when you assist the dental officer in treating a patient.

The first section of this chapter deals with the anatomy of the head and neck. When you complete the section, you should be able to identify the major bones of the cranium and face, the anatomical landmarks of the maxillae and the mandible, the muscles of mastication, and the structures of the respiratory system located in the head and neck. The second section of the chapter covers dental anatomy, providing a description of the external features of the teeth. When you finish the section, you should be able to identify these features and classify each tooth by name, location, and number. Upon completing the final section, "Dental Histology," you should be able to identify the tissues of the teeth and their supporting structures.

This chapter contains many new, unfamiliar words. Therefore, when you read the chapter, you may want to refer to
a glossary that defines some commonly used medical and dental terms. You should become familiar with such terms.

1. ANATOMY OF THE HEAD AND NECK

The dental assistant is concerned not only with the teeth themselves, but also with their surrounding tissues and supporting structures. The major bones of the skull form supporting structures for the teeth and provide attachments for many of the muscles responsible for the masticatory (chewing) process. Some of these bones actually form the sockets in which the teeth are embedded. The skull is composed of cranial bones and facial bones.

CRANIAL BONES

The cranium, which encases and protects the brain, consists of eight bones: the frontal bone, two temporal bones, two parietal bones, the occipital bone, the sphenoid bone, and the ethmoid bone (figs. 1 and 2). The sphenoid and ethmoid bones are not important to the present study, so they are not discussed here, nor are they shown in the figures.

The frontal bone forms the forehead, part of the roof of the eye sockets, and part of the nasal cavity. The frontal sinuses (air spaces in the bone) are located above each eye socket.

One temporal bone is located on each side of the skull. These bones form part of the sides and the base of the skull in the area of the ears. The bones house the hearing organs.

The two parietal bones are located posteriorly to (behind) the frontal bone. The parietal bones form the greater part of the roof and the sides of the skull.

The occipital bone forms the back and part of the base of the skull. There is a large foramen, or opening, in this bone through which the spinal cord passes.

FACIAL BONES

The facial bones include two each of the following: the nasal bones, the inferior nasal conchae, the lacrimal bones, the zygomatic bones, the palatine bones, and the maxillae; in addition, there is one vomer and one mandible (figs. 1 and 2). Some of these bones—the lacrimal bones, the inferior nasal conchae, and the vomer—are unimportant to the present study, so they are not discussed here, nor are they shown in the figures.

The nasal bones are small and oblong. They are located side by side at the middle and upper part of the nose. When they are joined, these bones form the upper part of the bridge of the nose.

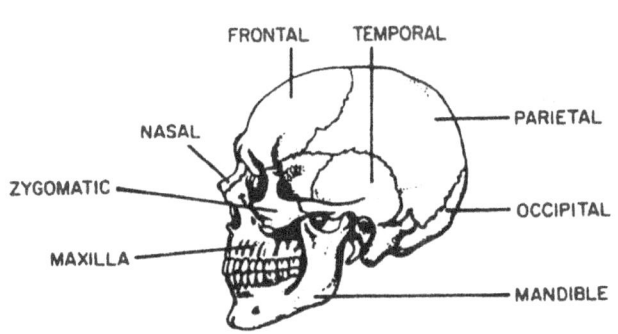

Figure 1.—The skull, side view.

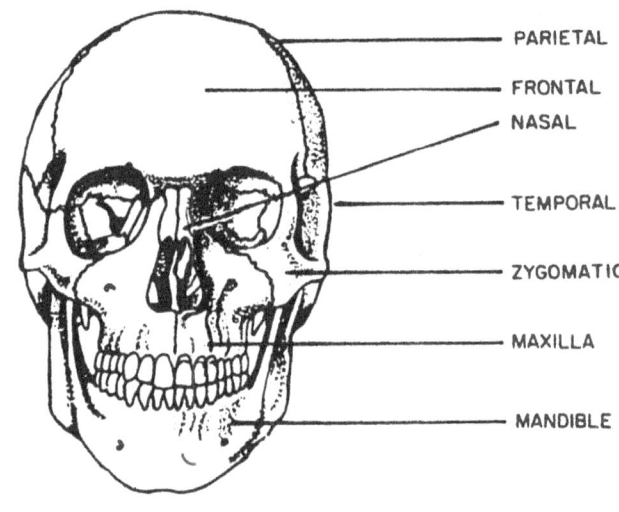

Figure 2.—The skull, front view.

The zygomatic bones, or "cheekbones," form the prominent part of the cheek under each eye.

The palatine bones form the right and left posterior portions of the palate, or roof of the mouth (fig. 3). They also contribute to the formation of the floor and the outer walls of the nasal cavity.

Of all the facial bones, the most important for dentistry are the maxillae and the mandible. Following is a discussion of the major features (landmarks) of these facial bones.

DENTAL FUNDAMENTALS

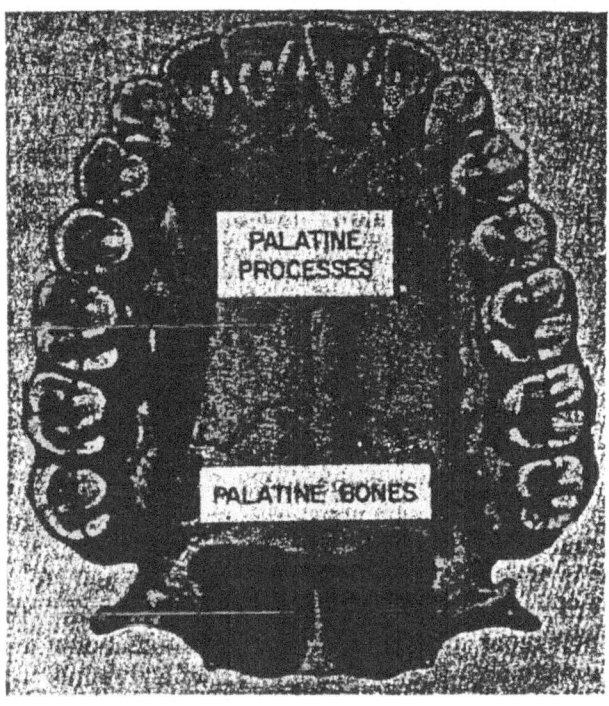

Figure 3.—The palate, showing the palatine bones and the palatine processes.

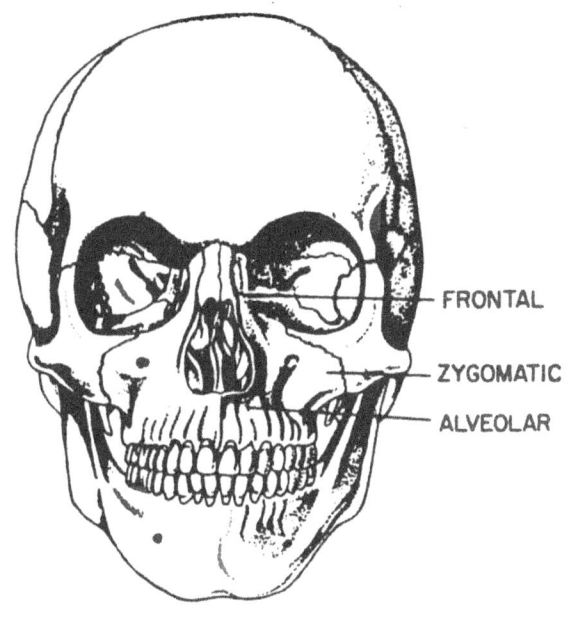

Figure 4.—The frontal, zygomatic, and alveolar processes of the maxilla.

Landmarks of the Maxillae

The maxillae (plural, maxilla is singular) are two facial bones that unite to form the upper jaw. Each maxilla contributes to the formation of the boundaries of the roof of the mouth, the floor and the outer walls of the nose, and the floor of each eye socket.

Each maxilla has a body and four processes. The body is shaped like a pyramid, and within the walls of the body is a large cavity—the maxillary sinus—which is the largest sinus in the skull. The four processes located on each maxilla are the frontal, zygomatic, alveolar, and palatine (figs. 3 and 4).

The frontal process extends upward and backward along the side of the nose. The zygomatic process joins the zygomatic bone to form the zygomatic arch, which makes up the foundation of the cheek. The alveolar process extends downward from the body of each maxilla to provide eight deep sockets into which fit the roots of teeth. When the right and left maxillae are united, the alveolar processes form the maxillary arch. The palatine processes unite to form the roof of the mouth and the anterior (front) portion of the floor of the nasal cavity.

Landmarks of the Mandible

The mandible, or lower jawbone, is a single bone consisting of a horizontal body, curved somewhat in the manner of a horseshoe, and two rami (plural, ramus is singular) that rise perpendicular to the body (fig. 5). The alveolar process of the mandible, like the alveolar processes of the maxillae, contains sockets for the roots of teeth.

The upper border of each ramus presents two distinct features: the coronoid process and the condyloid process. The coronoid process is the anterior projection of each ramus. It serves as an attachment for the muscle that raises the mandible. The condyloid process, or condyle, is the posterior projection of each ramus. It forms a hinge joint with a socket in the temporal bone. This joint is referred to as the temporomandibular joint. It is because of this joint that the mandible is able to move independently of the maxillae.

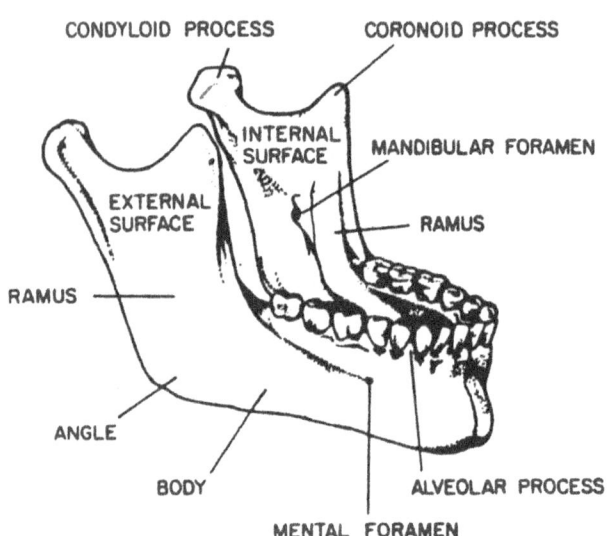

Figure 5.—The mandible.

On the internal surface of each ramus is the mandibular foramen, which provides an entrance for blood vessels and nerves. The nerves and blood vessels continue through the body of the mandible, exiting on the external surface of the mandible at the mental foramen (one is located on each side of the mandible). At the lower junction of the body and the ramus is located the angle of the mandible.

MUSCLES OF MASTICATION

The movement of the mandible is controlled by four pairs of muscles: the masseter, temporalis, medial pterygoid, and lateral pterygoid muscles. Taken together, these four pairs of muscles are known as the major muscles of mastication. Each of these major muscles of mastication will be discussed in terms of origin, insertion, and action.

Each muscle has two ends. One end is called the origin, the other the insertion. The origin is the end of the muscle that is attached to a relatively fixed part of the skeleton; thus, the origin remains more or less stationary when the muscle contracts. The insertion, on the other hand, is the end of the muscle that is attached to a more movable part of the skeleton; thus, the insertion shows more movement than the origin when the muscle contracts. The action of a muscle is the movement of organs or parts of the body produced by the muscle when it contracts.

Masseter muscle:—This is a flat, thick muscle that originates along the zygomatic arch and inserts into the lateral surfaces of the angle and ramus of the mandible (fig. 6). The action of the muscle is to raise the mandible and close the mouth.

Temporalis muscle:—This is a large, fan-shaped muscle that originates along the temporal bone and inserts into the coronoid process of the mandible (fig. 6). The action of this muscle is to assist the masseter muscle in raising the mandible and closing the mouth.

Medial pterygoid muscle:—This is a triheaded muscle that originates on the pterygoid process of the sphenoid bone and inserts into the medial surface of the ramus (fig. 7). The action of the muscle is to raise the mandible and close the mouth.

Lateral pterygoid muscle:—This is a biheaded muscle that originates on the pterygoid process of the sphenoid bone and inserts into the

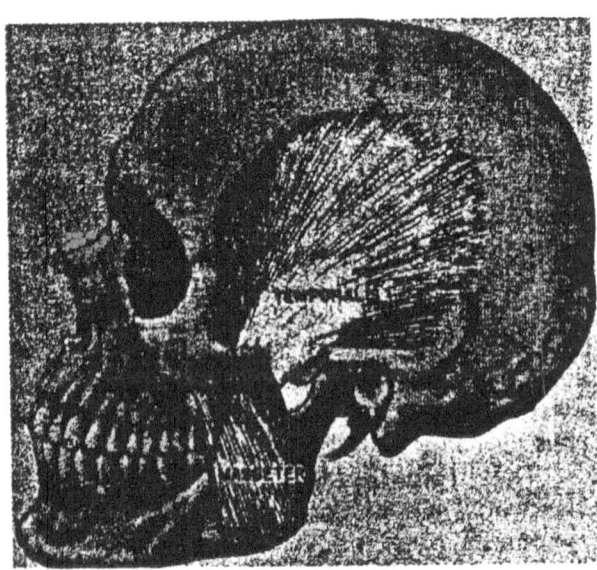

Figure 6.—Masseter and temporalis muscles.

DENTAL FUNDAMENTALS

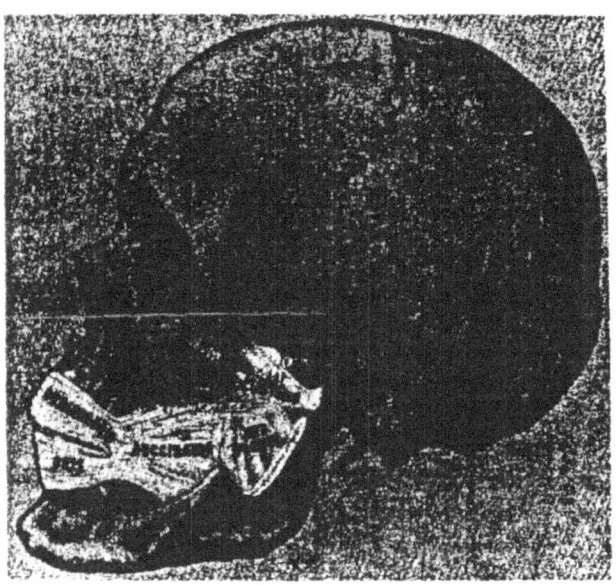

Figure 7.—Medial and lateral pterygoid, buccinator, and orbicularis oris muscles.

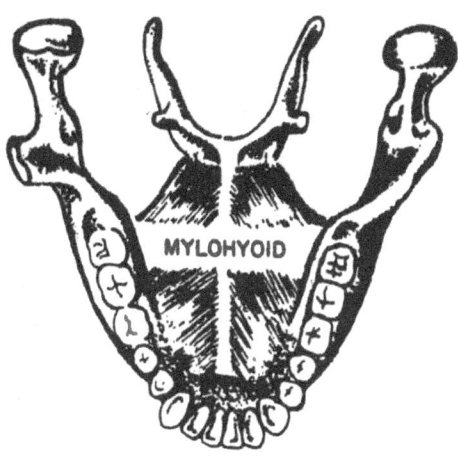

Figure 8.—The mylohyoid muscle.

condyloid process of the mandible (fig. 7). In mastication, this muscle acts to protrude or depress the mandible (open the mouth).

Acting independently, but always in association with the major muscles of mastication, are several accessory muscles of mastication. The buccinator muscle forms the cheek, and the orbicularis oris muscle forms the lips (fig. 7). The mylohyoid muscle forms the floor of the mouth under the tongue (fig. 8). The tongue itself is a muscular organ that moves food around in the mouth and aids in mastication.

STRUCTURES OF THE RESPIRATORY SYSTEM

Respiration (breathing) is one of the vital functions of the body. The dental assistant should have a basic understanding of the respiratory structures, since he may be required to perform emergency resuscitative procedures in the dental operatory.

Respiration causes air to be drawn into and expelled from the lungs. Respiration provides oxygen for the body tissues and serves as the main exhaust for carbon dioxide. The following paragraphs describe the path of the air as it enters the nose and mouth until it passes into the lungs, where a transfer of oxygen and carbon dioxide takes place. Figure 9 shows the major respiratory structures involved in this process.

The air enters the nasal cavity through the nostrils. Lining the nasal passages are tiny hairs called cilia. These hairs, along with mucous membranes, trap and filter out dust and other minute particles of foreign matter. In the chambers of the nasal cavity, the air is warmed and moistened. The air then passes through the pharynx, which is the upper part of the throat. The pharynx is a passageway for both food and air; it also filters the air before the air goes any farther.

The air next passes through the larynx, or "voice box," which is located between the base of the tongue and the trachea. It is here that the vocal cords are found. The larynx is covered by a flap of tissue, the epiglottis. When a person swallows, the epiglottis covers the entrance of the larynx, preventing foods or liquids from entering the trachea. After the air has passed through the larynx, it enters the trachea, or windpipe. The trachea is a tube lined with cilia and mucous membranes for filtration. The trachea carries the air to the lungs, where the transfer of oxygen and carbon dioxide occurs.

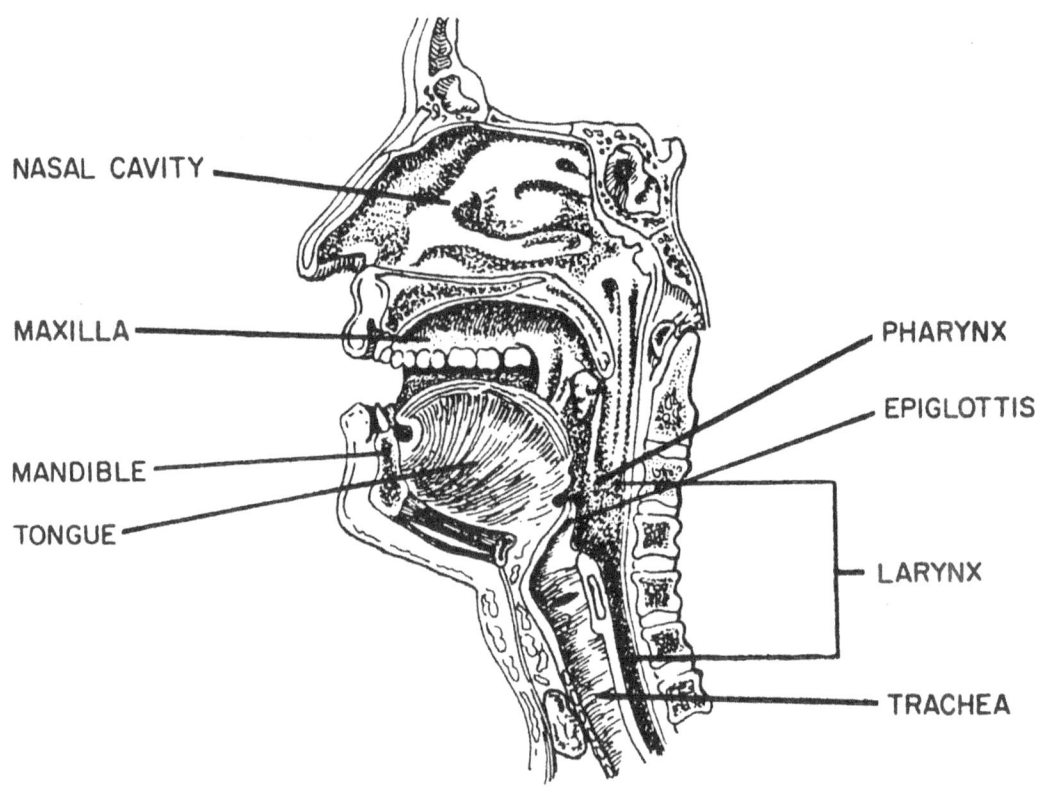

Figure 9.—Structures of the respiratory system.

2. DENTAL ANATOMY

Dental anatomy deals with the external features of the teeth. To understand the material in this section, you must become familiar with the terms used to describe the external features of the teeth. To perform your duties efficiently and completely, you must know the full name, the location, and the anatomy of each tooth in the mouth. In addition, you must know the numbering system by which the teeth are identified on the standard dental chart used by the armed services. Such knowledge will be useful to you throughout your career, when you fill in dental charts, expose radiographs, clean teeth, and assist in all phases of dentistry.

In the discussion that follows, keep in mind that teeth differ in size, shape, and other characteristics from one person to another. This discussion concentrates on the most commonly observed external features of the teeth.

FUNCTIONS OF THE TEETH

Each tooth in the mouth can be classified as either an incisor, a cuspid, a bicuspid, or a molar (fig. 10). Each type of tooth performs a particular function in the masticatory process. The incisors have edges for cutting food. The cuspids and bicuspids have points (cusps) for grasping and tearing food. The molars have broad chewing surfaces for grinding solid masses of food.

LOCATION OF THE TEETH

Normally, the adult human gets two sets of teeth during his lifetime. The first (deciduous) set consists of 20 teeth. The second (permanent) set usually consists of 32 teeth. Half of the teeth are located in the maxillary arch, embedded in the alveolar processes of the maxillae. These are the maxillary teeth. The remaining half of the teeth are located in the mandibular arch,

DENTAL FUNDAMENTALS

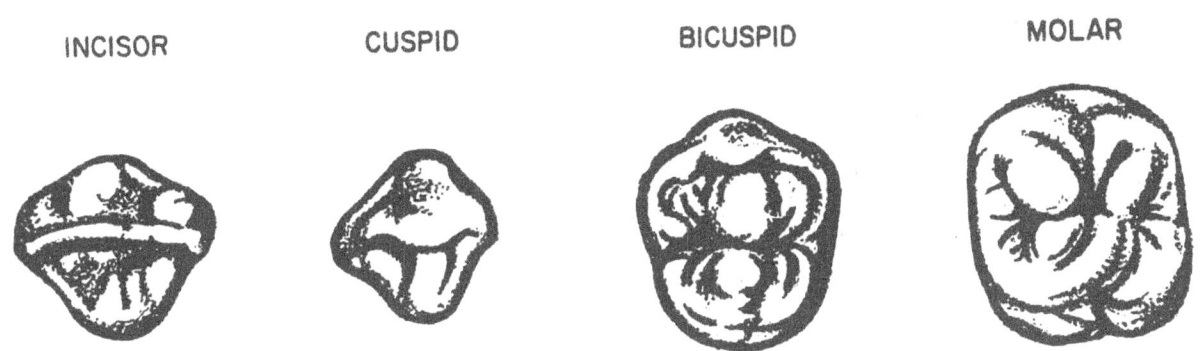

Figure 10.—Types of human teeth.

embedded in the alveolar process of the mandible. These are the mandibular teeth.

The mouth is divided into two arches, the maxillary arch and the mandibular arch. Each arch, in turn, is divided into a right and a left quadrant. The quadrants are formed by an imaginary line called the midline, or median line, that passes between the central incisors in each arch and divides the arch in half (fig. 11). There are four quadrants in the mouth (two per arch), and they divide the mouth into four equal parts. (Quadrant means "one fourth," and each quadrant is one fourth of the entire mouth.) Teeth are described as being located in one of the four quadrants: the right maxillary quadrant, the left maxillary quadrant, the right mandibular quadrant, or the left mandibular quadrant.

In each quadrant, there are eight permanent teeth: two incisors, one cuspid, two bicuspids, and three molars (fig. 12). The tooth positioned immediately to the side of the midline is the central incisor, so called because it occupies a central location in the arch. To the side of the central incisor is the lateral incisor. Next is the cuspid, then the two bicuspids (the first bicuspid, followed by the second bicuspid). The last teeth are the molars. There are three molars. After the second bicuspid comes the first molar, followed by the second molar, followed by the third molar (the "wisdom tooth").

Another, but less exact, method of describing the location of the teeth is to refer to them as anterior or posterior teeth (fig. 12). Anterior teeth are those located in the front of the mouth, the incisors and the cuspids. Normally, these are the teeth that are visible when a person smiles. The posterior teeth are those located in the back of the mouth, the bicuspids and the molars.

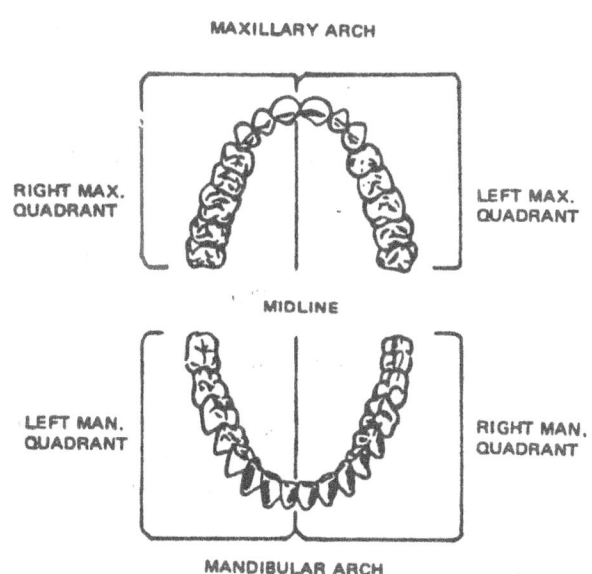

Figure 11.—Maxillary and mandibular arches divided into quadrants.

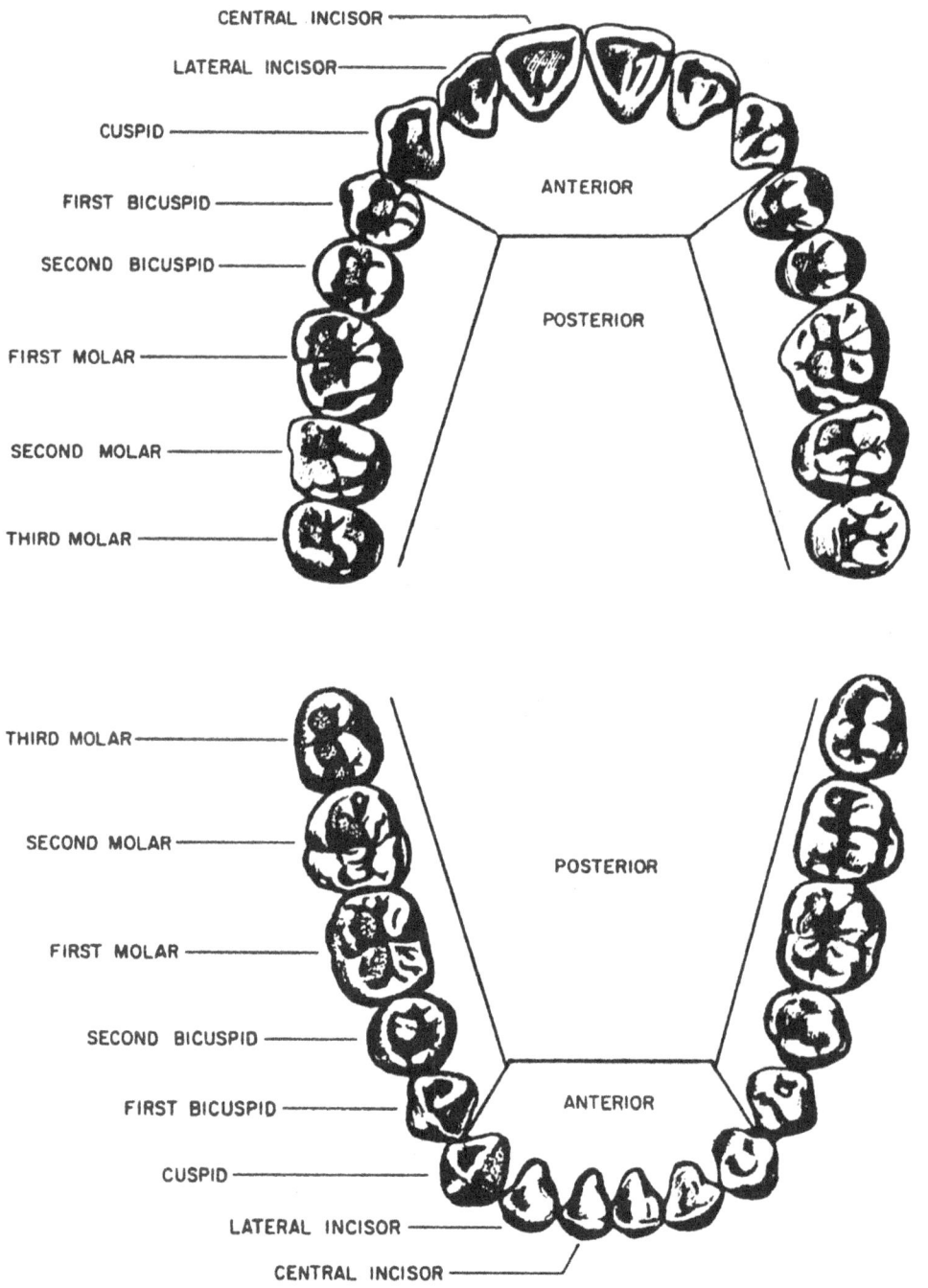

Figure 12.—Names of the teeth in the right maxillary and mandibular quadrants; anterior and posterior teeth.

DENTAL FUNDAMENTALS

IDENTIFICATION OF THE TEETH

In order to avoid confusion, you must identify a tooth as completely as possible. Give its full name: central incisor (not just incisor), second molar (not just molar), etc. But even the full name of a tooth does not provide adequate identification, since there are several teeth with the same name. Complete tooth identification requires that you identify the quadrant in which the tooth appears, in addition to giving the full name of the tooth. Therefore, you would identify a specific second molar in the following manner: right mandibular second molar. Although there are four second molars in the mouth, naming the quadrant (right mandibular) narrows the field down to one specific second molar.

There is a simplified method of identifying the teeth. This method employs numbers, with each tooth designated by a separate number from 1 to 32. Although there are several accepted numbering systems, only the one used by the armed services will be explained here. Figure 13 shows the numbering system employed on the standard dental chart. When charting, you would refer to a tooth by number rather than name. Instead of referring to the right maxillary third molar, you would refer to tooth No. 1. Each tooth has its own number. If any tooth is missing from the mouth, always leave a space for it when counting the teeth. For example, if the

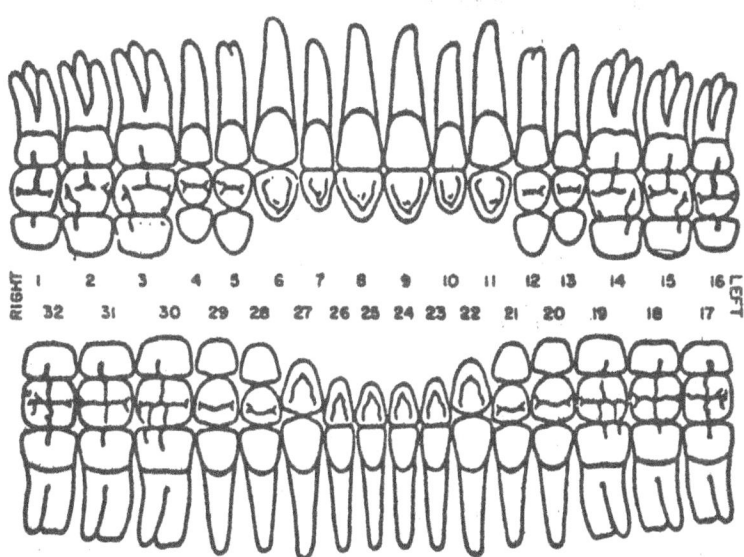

1. Right maxillary third molar.
2. Right maxillary second molar.
3. Right maxillary first molar.
4. Right maxillary second bicuspid.
5. Right maxillary first bicuspid.
6. Right maxillary cuspid.
7. Right maxillary lateral incisor.
8. Right maxillary central incisor.
9. Left maxillary central incisor.
10. Left maxillary lateral incisor.
11. Left maxillary cuspid.
12. Left maxillary first bicuspid.
13. Left maxillary second bicuspid.
14. Left maxillary first molar.
15. Left maxillary second molar.
16. Left maxillary third molar.
17. Left mandibular third molar.
18. Left mandibular second molar.
19. Left mandibular first molar.
20. Left mandibular second bicuspid.
21. Left mandibular first bicuspid.
22. Left mandibular cuspid.
23. Left mandibular lateral incisor.
24. Left mandibular central incisor.
25. Right mandibular central incisor.
26. Right mandibular lateral incisor.
27. Right mandibular cuspid.
28. Right mandibular first bicuspid.
29. Right mandibular second bicuspid.
30. Right mandibular first molar.
31. Right mandibular second molar.
32. Right mandibular third molar.

Figure 13.—Standard dental chart; names and numbers of the teeth.

right maxillary second molar (No. 2) is missing, the right maxillary first molar still remains tooth No. 3, the right maxillary second bicuspid No. 4, and so on. Failure to follow this procedure will cause confusion and result in misnumbering the teeth.

When using the standard dental chart, remember that the right and left sides are reversed. The right side of a patient's mouth appears on the left side of the dental chart; the left side of a patient's mouth appears on the right side of the dental chart. (The directional terms "left" and "right" are printed on the chart to avoid confusion.) This arrangement is necessary because the dental officer and the assistant see the sides reversed when they look into a patient's mouth.

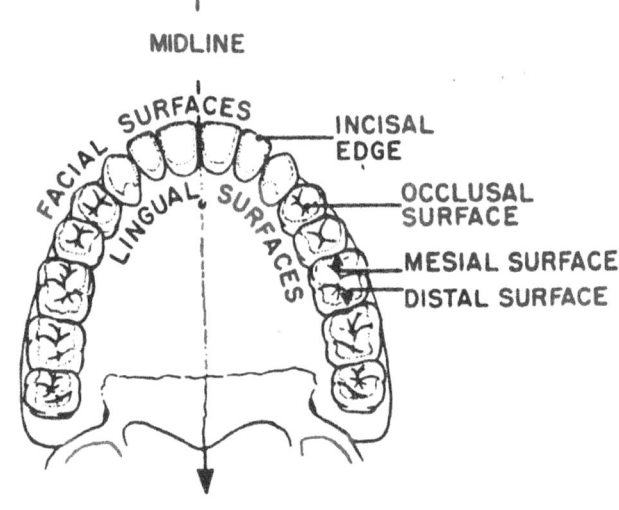

Figure 14.—Surfaces of the teeth.

SURFACES OF THE TEETH

Not only must the assistant be able to name and locate a tooth, but he must also be able to identify a specific tooth surface. Figure 14 shows a number of the different surfaces of the teeth.

The facial surface is the outer surface of a tooth adjacent to the lips and the cheeks. The facial surface of an anterior tooth is often referred to as the labial surface because it lies next to the labia, or lips. The facial surface of a posterior tooth is often referred to as the buccal surface because it lies next to the buccinator, or cheek, muscle.

The lingual surface is the surface of an anterior or posterior tooth that faces toward the tongue.

The mesial surface is the surface of a tooth that, following the curvature of the dental arch, is closest to or facing the midline of the arch.

Distal is the opposite of mesial. The distal surface is the tooth surface that, following the curvature of the dental arch, faces away from the midline.

Incisal edges are narrow cutting edges found only on the anterior teeth (incisors and cuspids). Incisors have one incisal edge. Cuspids have two incisal edges that meet at the tip of the cusp.

The occlusal surface is the broad chewing surface found on posterior teeth (bicuspids and molars).

To get a clearer picture of the various tooth surfaces, refer to figure 13, which has previously been discussed. The standard dental chart shows each of the teeth "unfolded," so that the facial, occlusal or incisal, and lingual surfaces of the teeth can be shown. For the posterior teeth, the facial surfaces are shown adjacent to the roots, followed by the occlusal surfaces, and then by the lingual surfaces (which are located next to the numbers on the chart). For the anterior teeth, the facial surfaces are shown adjacent to the roots, and the incisal edges are shown as a line between the facial and lingual surfaces. The lingual surfaces are located next to the numbers on the chart.

Tooth surfaces that face each other are called proximal surfaces (fig. 15). The proximal surface includes the entire length of the tooth from the crown to the root tip. The point on proximal surfaces where two teeth actually touch each other is the contact point. The area between the teeth is referred to as the interproximal space. Part of the interproximal space is occupied by the interdental papilla (singular, papillae is plural). The interdental papilla is a triangular fold of gingival tissue. The

DENTAL FUNDAMENTALS

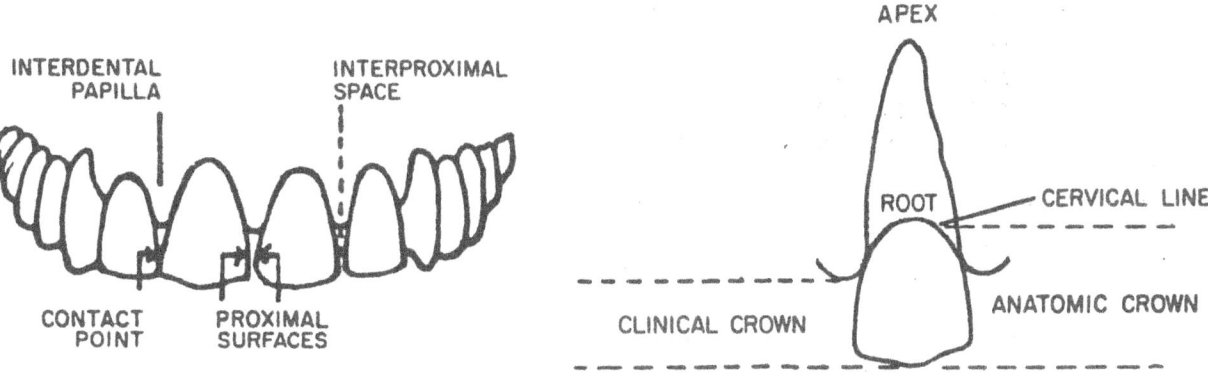

Figure 15.—Adjacent tooth surfaces and spaces.

Figure 17.—Tooth crown and root.

part of the interproximal space not occupied by the interdental papilla is called the embrasure. The embrasure occupies an area bordered by the interdental papilla, the proximal surfaces of two adjacent teeth, and the contact point (fig. 16). If there is no contact point between the teeth, then the area between them is called a diastema instead of an embrasure.

ANATOMICAL LANDMARKS

Every tooth has a crown and a root portion (fig. 17). The crown is divided into the anatomic crown and the clinical crown. The anatomic crown is the part of the tooth that is covered with enamel. The clinical crown is the part of the tooth that is exposed (visible) in the mouth. The cervical line, or cervix, is a slight indentation that encircles the tooth and marks the junction of the crown with the root. The tip of each root is called the apex. On the apex of each root, there is a small opening that allows for the passage of blood vessels and nerves into the tooth. This opening is called the apical foramen.

A tooth may have a single root or it may have two, three, or more. When a tooth has two roots, the root portion is said to be bifurcated. When it has three roots, the root portion is said to be trifurcated (fig. 18). If a tooth has four or more roots, it is said to be multirooted. As a general rule, maxillary molars have three roots

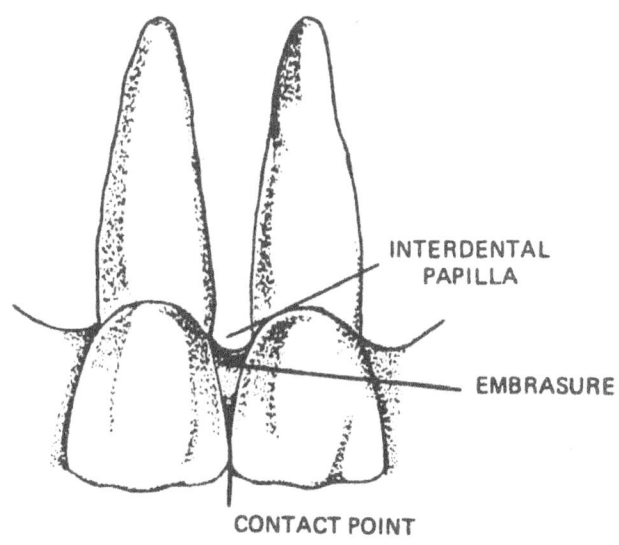

Figure 16.—Embrasure.

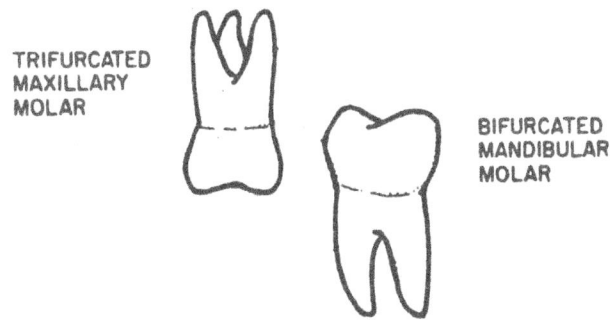

Figure 18.—Trifurcated and bifurcated roots.

and mandibular molars have two roots. Most bicuspids are single rooted, although approximately 50 percent of maxillary first bicuspids are bifurcated at the apex. Anterior teeth are single rooted.

A cusp is a rounded point on the working surface of a cuspid, bicuspid, or molar. A cuspid has a single cusp, a bicuspid has two, and a molar has four (sometimes five) cusps. If a fifth cusp is found, it will be on a maxillary first molar, usually on the lingual surface of the mesiolingual cusp. This fifth cusp is called the cusp of Carabelli. Figure 19 shows the significant features of the occlusal surface of a maxillary first molar.

A ridge is a linear elevation on the surface of a tooth. Several different ridges can be found on a tooth. A marginal ridge is the elevation of enamel that forms the mesial and distal margins (edges) of a tooth. On posterior teeth, this ridge is on the occlusal surfaces; on anterior teeth, it can be found on the lingual surfaces. A transverse ridge is any ridge found on posterior teeth that crosses the occlusal surface between cusps. This ridge is not shown in figure 19; it is most prominent on maxillary bicuspids. An oblique ridge is found only on maxillary first and second molars. It crosses the occlusal surface diagonally from the distofacial cusp to the mesiolingual cusp. You should remember the location of this ridge. It is important for charting and for operative dentistry, since the dentist tries to preserve this strong ridge whenever possible.

A groove is a linear depression on the surface of a tooth. A marginal groove is a depression running perpendicular to a marginal ridge. Facial and lingual grooves are, simply, grooves on the facial and lingual surfaces of the teeth. Usually, they are extensions of a groove on the occlusal surface. The central groove is a depression passing from the mesial to the distal marginal ridges on the occlusal surface of a bicuspid. Grooves are indicated on the standard dental chart by means of dark lines (fig. 13).

A fossa is a shallow, irregular depression on the surface of a tooth. A pit is a small, definite pinpoint depression on the surface of a tooth. It is usually found at the bottom of a fossa, at the junction of two or more grooves, or at the end of a facial or lingual groove.

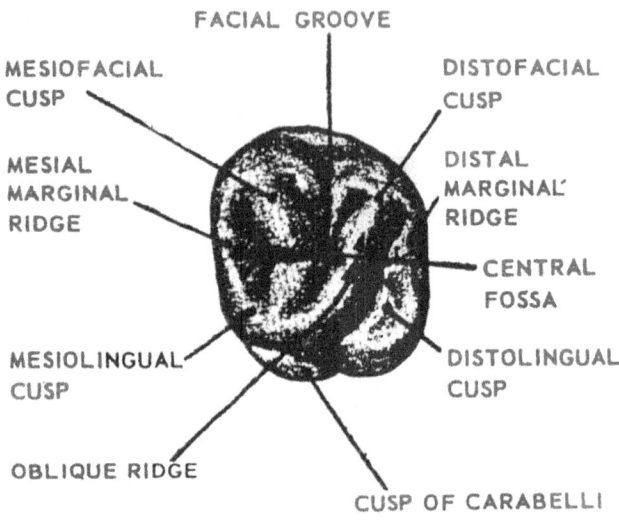

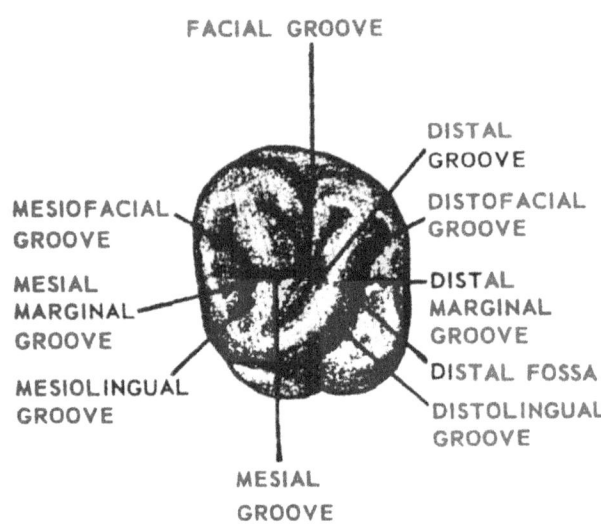

Figure 19.—Features of the occlusal surface of a maxillary first molar.

OCCLUSAL RELATIONSHIPS

Occlusion is the relationship between the occlusal surfaces of opposing maxillary and mandibular teeth when the teeth are in contact. When the mouth is closed and there is maximum contact between the occlusal surfaces of the mandibular and maxillary teeth, the position is

DENTAL FUNDAMENTALS

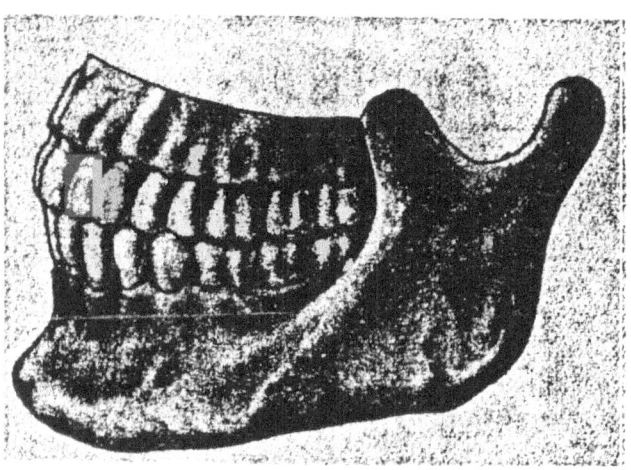

Figure 20.—Centric occlusion.

called centric occlusion (fig. 20). In normal jaw relations, when the teeth are of normal size and in the correct position, the mesiofacial cusp of the maxillary first molar fits into the facial groove of the mandibular first molar. This relationship between the two teeth is called the key to occlusion. The key to occlusion is clinical evidence of the correct relationship of the mandible to the maxillae.

The term "malocclusion" is used to describe any deviation from normal occlusion. Vertical overlap, or overbite, is a condition in which the vertical distance between the maxillary and mandibular incisal edges is abnormal when the other teeth are in normal occlusion (fig. 21).

Horizontal overlap, also called overjet or buck teeth, is a condition in which the horizontal distance between the maxillary and mandibular incisal edges is abnormal when the other teeth are in normal occlusion (fig. 21).

A prognathic maxillomandibular relationship is a condition in which there is a marked projection of the mandible, usually resulting in the lower teeth hitting anterior to the maxillary incisors (fig. 22). A retrognathic maxillomandibular relationship is a condition in which there is a marked recession of the mandible, producing a very receding chin (fig. 23).

3. DENTAL HISTOLOGY

Dental anatomy deals with the external form and appearance of the teeth. Dental histology

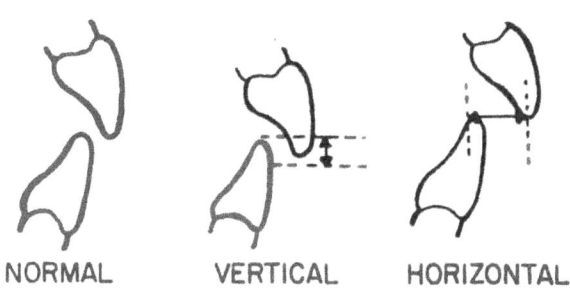

Figure 21.—Normal occlusion; vertical and horizontal overlap.

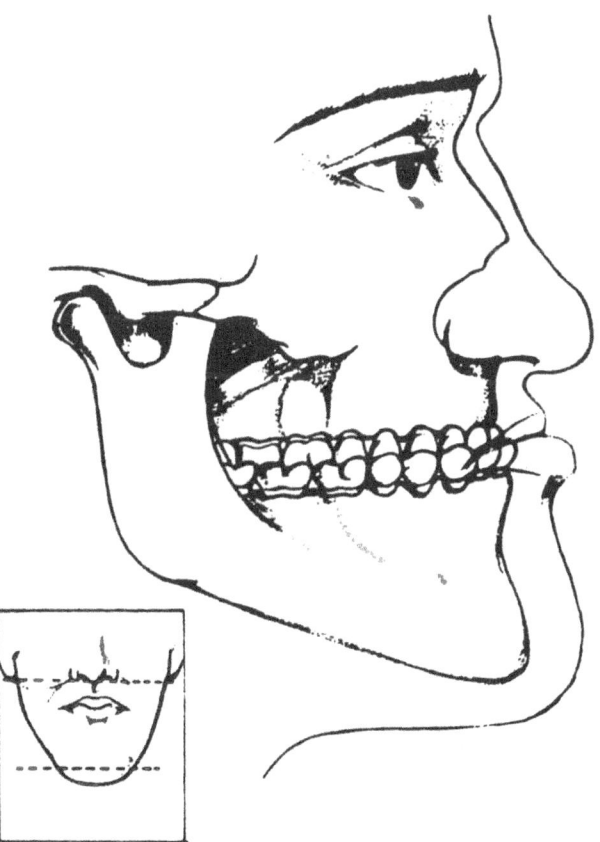

Figure 22.—Prognathic maxillomandibular relationship.

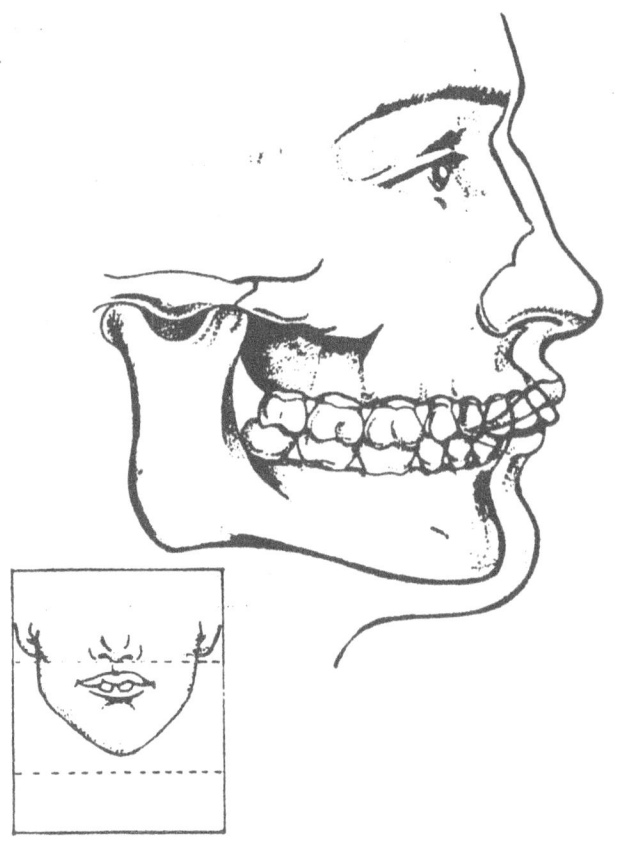

Figure 23.—Retrognathic maxillomandibular relationship.

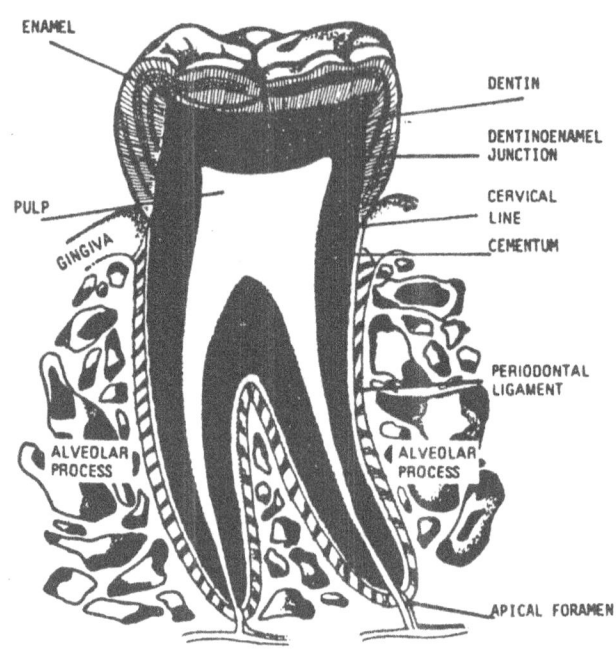

Figure 24.—The periodontium.

studies the tissues and internal structure of the teeth, along with the tissues that surround and support the teeth (tissues of the periodontium). A knowledge of dental histology will be of help to you when you mount radiographs, clean teeth, and provide emergency dental treatment.

TISSUES OF THE TEETH

Structurally, the teeth are composed of four different tissues: enamel, dentin, cementum, and pulp (fig. 24). Cementum is also considered a tissue of the periodontium, since it supports the teeth by providing attachment for the principal fibers of the periodontal ligament.

Enamel

Enamel is the calcified substance that covers the entire crown of the tooth. It consists of approximately 96 percent inorganic (nonliving) material, and it is the hardest tissue in the human body. Enamel is thickest at the cusps, thinning to a knife edge at the cervical line. The color of a tooth is derived from the enamel, which is usually shaded from light yellow to white.

Enamel is formed by cells called ameloblasts. Enamel is completely formed prior to tooth eruption, after which the ameloblasts become nonfunctional. This means that enamel is formed only once and cannot regenerate or repair itself. Thus, when enamel is destroyed by decay, operative dentistry is required to reconstruct the tooth. Enamel has no nerve fibers and cannot register sensations. It is strong and hard; it has the ability to withstand masticating forces; it resists abrasion or attrition; and it is thick in areas that contact opposing teeth. Because of these properties, enamel serves to protect the underlying softer dentin.

Dentin

Dentin is the light yellow substance that makes up the bulk of the tooth. Dentin is the

DENTAL FUNDAMENTALS

second hardest substance in the body. It is softer than enamel, but harder than bone. It consists of approximately 70 percent inorganic matter. It is slightly elastic and compressible.

Dentin is found inside the crown under the enamel. The point at which the dentin and the enamel meet is called the dentinoenamel junction. Dentin is also found inside the root of the tooth under the cementum. The inner surface of the dentin forms a hard-walled cavity that contains and protects the pulp.

Dentin is formed by cells called odontoblasts, which are part of the pulp. All of the dentin of a newly formed tooth is called primary dentin. Unlike enamel, dentin continues to form throughout the life of the tooth. When the dental pulp is mildly stimulated as a result of caries, cavity preparation, abrasion, attrition, or erosion, a protective layer of secondary dentin is formed on the pulp wall. When irritation is severe, irregular dentin is formed. Irregular dentin differs from secondary dentin only in that the irregular dentin is structurally weaker.

Even though dentin is not sensitive to stimuli, sensation may result when mechanical, thermal, or chemical stimuli are applied to the dentin. The sensation comes not from the dentin itself but from odontoblastic cells that extend into the dentin. These cells are actually part of the pulp, not the dentin, and they are sensitive to stimuli.

Cementum

Cementum is a bonelike substance, although it is not so hard as bone. It consists of approximately 50 percent inorganic material, and it forms a protective layer over the root portion of the dentin. The cementum joins the enamel at the cervix of the tooth. The point at which they join is called the cementoenamel junction (fig. 25). The cementum is thinnest at this junction. In most teeth, the cementum overlaps the enamel for a short distance. In some teeth, the cementum meets the enamel in a sharp line. In a few teeth, there is a break between the cementum and the enamel, exposing a narrow area of root dentin. Such areas are sensitive to thermal, chemical, or mechanical stimuli.

The main function of cementum is to anchor the tooth to the socket by providing attachment

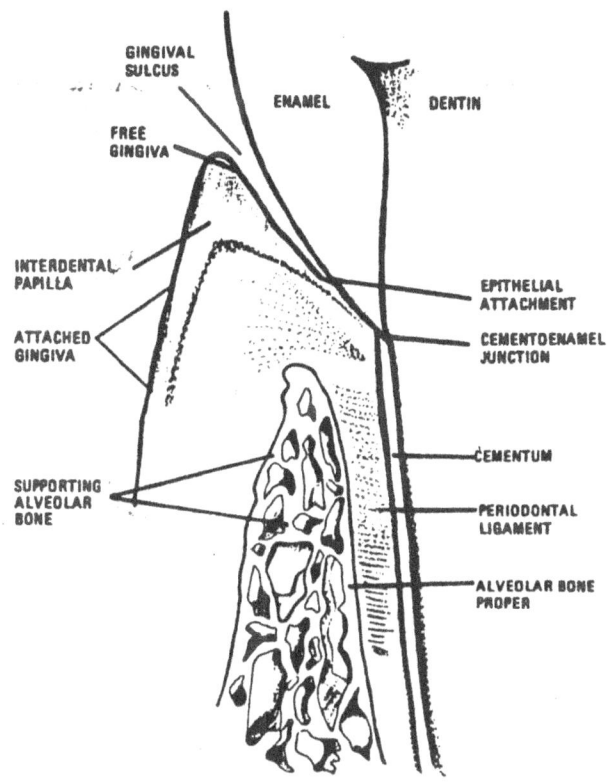

Figure 25.—Closeup view of the periodontium.

for the principal fibers of the periodontal ligament. (Additional information on this will be provided in the discussion of the periodontal ligament.) Cementum is formed continuously throughout the life of the tooth. Thus, it compensates for the loss of tooth substance due to occlusal wear, and it allows for the attachment of new fibers of the periodontal ligament to the root.

Pulp

The pulp is the soft tissue that fills the pulp cavity. This tissue contains numerous blood vessels and nerves which enter the tooth through the apical foramen. The pulp is enclosed within the hard, unyielding dentin walls of the pulp cavity. The pulp cavity has two parts: the pulp chamber and the root, or pulp, canal. The pulp chamber is located inside the crown. The root canal is located inside the root.

An important function of the pulp is the formation of dentin. The pulp provides the cells (odontoblasts) from which dentin is formed. The pulp also supplies the dentin with blood.

Pulp responds to external stimuli, providing sensation to the tooth. The pulp responds to irritation either by forming secondary dentin or by becoming inflamed. Since the walls of the pulp chamber and root canal permit no expansion of the pulp tissue, any inflammatory swelling of the tissue will compress the blood vessels against the walls. This results in a condition known as hyperemic pulp, which can lead to necrosis (death) of the pulp tissue.

TISSUES OF THE PERIODONTIUM

The tissues that surround and support the teeth are the cementum, the alveolar process, the periodontal ligament, and the gingiva. Collectively, these tissues are known as the periodontium. The cementum has been covered earlier, so it will not be discussed in this section. Throughout the following discussion, you should refer to figure 24 and to figure 25, which provides a closeup view of the periodontium.

Alveolar Process

The alveolar process is that portion of the maxillae and mandible that forms and supports the sockets (alveoli) of the teeth.

The alveolar process can be divided into two parts: the alveolar bone proper (or lamina dura) and the supporting alveolar bone. The alveolar bone proper is a thin layer of bone that lines the tooth socket and gives attachment to the principal fibers of the periodontal ligament. The supporting alveolar bone is the portion of the alveolar process that surrounds the alveolar bone proper and gives support to the tooth socket. The supporting alveolar bone is composed of inner and outer plates of compact bone (the cortical plates). Between these plates is found spongy, porous cancellous bone.

The quantity and quality of alveolar bone are affected by the amount of functional stress. If, because of tooth loss, a tooth in one arch does not make contact with any teeth in the opposing arch, the alveolar bone of the tooth socket will be under reduced stress and the bone will become much more rarefied (porous). When all the teeth are lost, the entire alveolar process undergoes partial atrophy.

Periodontal Ligament

The periodontal ligament consists of hundreds of tissue fibers that, except at the apical foramen, completely surround the root of the tooth. The ligament acts as a shock absorber, reducing the impact of the teeth as they occlude.

The periodontal ligament contains numerous bundles of fibers (principal fibers) that attach the tooth to the socket. These principal fibers are embedded on one side in the cementum of the tooth root and on the other side in the alveolar bone proper. In this manner, the tooth is suspended in the socket. Since the principal fibers are somewhat elastic, they permit a small amount of tooth movement. Also, the fibers are positioned so that the tooth can resist forces exerted upon it from all angles.

The periodontal ligament also supplies nutrition to the alveolar process. It supports and attaches the gingiva. It registers sensations of heat, cold, pressure, pain, and touch. Since the periodontal ligament can register such a wide range of sensations (as opposed to the pulp, which registers only pain), it is of special diagnostic importance to the dental officer.

The periodontal ligament varies in thickness according to the person, the location of the tooth, and the amount of tooth function. In dental radiographs, the ligament appears as a thin, dark line around the root. The alveolar bone proper appears as a thin, white line around the ligament.

Gingiva

The gingiva (singular, gingivae is plural) is the soft tissue that covers the alveolar process and surrounds the necks of the teeth. The gingiva consists of an outer layer of epithelium and an inner layer of connective tissue.

Depending upon whether or not it is attached to the tooth, the gingiva is described as being free or attached. The free gingiva is that portion of the gingiva surrounding the neck of the tooth just above the cervix, not directly

DENTAL FUNDAMENTALS

attached to the tooth, and forming the soft tissue wall of the gingival sulcus. The gingival sulcus is the V-shaped space between the free gingiva and the tooth. It extends to a depth of approximately 2 mm, at which point the gingiva is attached to the tooth by the epithelial attachment. The interdental papilla is the portion of the gingiva that fills the interproximal space between two adjacent teeth. It consists of both free and attached gingiva.

A healthy gingiva is pink, firm, and resilient. It has a stippled appearance. Stippling refers to the "orange peel" texture of the healthy tissue. Inflammation causes a loss of stippling. When inflamed, the gingiva may become sore and swollen, and it may bleed.

GLOSSARY OF DENTAL SCIENCE

CONTENTS

	Page
Abrasion ...... Arch, dental	1
Artery ...... Cementocyte	2
Cementoenamel junction ..... Ectoderm	3
Edentulous .... Follicle, dental	
Fontanelles) .... Interdentale, superior	5
Interproximal ...... Mitosis	6
Model ...... Pedodontics	7
Periapical ...... Pulp chamber	8
Pulp, dental ...... Surface, lingual	9
Surface, occlusal ..... Zygomaxillare	10

GLOSSARY OF DENTAL SCIENCE

Abrasion Wear of the surfaces of the teeth as a result of their use in mastication. The condition to which the term is applied is usually a wear of abnormal amount which does not represent a corresponding abnormal use, the excessive wear being due to some unknown influence. (3)

Abscess A collection of pus in a cavity formed within the tissues of the body. (3)

Accelerator Anything which hastens a chemical or physical reaction. (3)

Accretion Addition by growth, or by deposit, little by little; may be either amorphous; i.e., leaving no lines showing the form of growth; or stratified, showing lines of increase. (3)

Acid, deoxyribonucleic (abbrev. DNA) A nucleic acid originally isolated from fish sperm and thymus gland, but later found in all living cells; on hydrolysis it yields adenine, guanine, cytosine, thymine, deoxyribose, and phosphoric acid; it carries the genetic code. (2)

Adhesion The union of substances that differ in their nature, as, adhesion of glue to wood, paste to paper, etc. To unite bodies by their surfaces. (3)

Alloy, n. A metallic material composed of two or more metals. (3)

Alloy, v. The act of compounding an alloy. (3)

Alloy, amalgam The metallic substance in the form of shavings, filings, or pellets, which is mixed with mercury to form a dental amalgam. (3)

Alloy, gold (dental) An alloy in which the principal ingredient is gold. (1)

Amalgam An alloy, one of the constituents of which is mercury. Silver and tin are the most common additional components of dental amalgam. (3)

Ameloblasts Enamel-forming cells.

Amylase Any one of a series of enzymes which convert starch into sugar.

Amylose 1. Any carbohyrate of the starch group; a polysaccharide. 2. The soluble constituent of starch. (2)

Amorphous Having no definite form; shapeless; not crystallized. (2)

Anastomose To communicate with one another, as arteries and veins.

Anchorage The points of fixation of dental fillings, or artificial crowns or bridges. (2)

Apatite A series of minerals of the general formula $3Ca_3(PO_4)_2 \cdot CaF_2$. (2)

Apex The terminal end of a cone; a conical end. The terminal end of a root of a tooth. (3)

Apical Pertaining to the apex or conical endings of the roots of teeth. (3)

Arch An arc or portion of a circle. Any object in nature or art which is curved, like an arc. The dental arch, the arrangement of the teeth in a bow shape or arc. Often means the jawbone together with the teeth it supports. (3)

Arch(es), branchial Four pairs of mesenchymal and later cartilaginous arches of the embryo in the region of the neck.

Arch, dental The curving structure formed by the crowns of the teeth in their normal position, or by the residual ridge after loss of the teeth. The inferior dental arch, or arch of the mandible, is formed by the lower teeth, and the superior dental arch, or arch of the maxilla, is formed by the upper teeth. (3)

Artery A blood vessel through which the blood passes from the heart to the various structures of the body. There are three layers of tissue in every artery: an inner coat (tunica intima), a middle coat (tunica media), and an outer coat (tunica adventitia). The structure of the three layers varies with the location, the size, and the function of the vessel.

Articular eminence See *Eminence, articular*.

Articulation The state of being joined together by a joint or joints. (2)

Articulation, temporomandibular The joint formed by the mandibular condyle of the lower jaw and the glenoid fossa of the skull. The articulation of the condyloid process of the mandible and the interarticular disk with the mandibular fossa of the temporal bone. (1)

Attrition The normal or abnormal loss of tooth structure due to friction caused by physiologic or pathologic forces interacting between the tooth and an abrasive substance, object, or other tooth or teeth. Also called abrasion. (1)

Basion The midline point on the brain capsule at the anterior margin of the occipital foramen.

BHN See *Brinell Hardness Number*.

Birefringent Doubly refractive. (2)

Bite The power of force with which the teeth may be closed in the crushing of food, is called the strength of the bite, or simply, the bite. It is measured with the gnathodynamometer. (3)

Bone The material of the skeleton of most vertebrate animals. It is derived from transformed mesenchymal cells enclosed in a ground substance containing connective tissue fibers. The ground substance, or bone matrix, is a hard, opaque, calcified material penetrated by bone vessels. The external surface is covered by a layer of dense connective tissue called the periosteum.

Bone, alveolar The portion of the alveolar process that surrounds the roots of the teeth. A thin plate of bone to which the periodontal ligament is attached. It is pierced by many small openings which transmit blood and lymph vessels and nerves to the periodontal ligament.

Bone, cancellous The bone that forms a trabecular network, surrounds marrow spaces that may contain either fatty or hematopoietic tissue, lies subjacent to the cortical bone, and makes up the main portion (bulk) of a bone. (1)

Bone, cortical The solid portion of the shaft of a bone which surrounds the medullary cavity. (2)

Bone, haversian Bone composed of haversian systems. (3)

Brain, capsule See *Capsule, brain*.

Bregma The point on the brain capsule at which sagittal and coronal sutures meet.

Brinell Hardness Number (abbr. BHN) A measure of hardness of a structure, obtained by determining the unit stress on the surface of an indentation made by a hardened steel ball of a specified diameter under a specified load. (3)

Brittleness, n. Lack of ability to withstand permanent deformation; lacking in plasticity; opposite of toughness. (3)

Bruxism The nonfunctional gnashing, grinding, or clenching of the teeth in sleep or, unconsciously, while awake. (1)

Buccal Pertaining to the cheek; toward the cheek; next to the cheek, etc. (3)

Bucco-lingual From the cheek toward the tongue; as the bucco-lingual diameter of the crown of a molar tooth. (3)

Calcification The act of depositing calcific matter or calcium salts during growth. The bones and teeth become calcified. Also pathological calcifications occur in several parts of the body. (3)

Calculus (calcareous deposit) Tartar, the mineral deposit on teeth. Bacteria of filamentous types appear to be an important constituent of calculus. Deposits of calculus may also form in salivary gland ducts, in the kidney, etc.

Canal A relatively narrow tubular passage or channel. (2)

Canal, haversian One of the freely anastomosing channels of the haversian system in compact bone. (2)

Canal, root The opening through the center of the long axis of the root of a tooth from the crown to the apex, which under normal conditions contains the root portion of the dental pulp.

Canaliculi dentales See *Tubules, dental*.

Capping A covering, as with a cap. A term applied to the operation of placing a covering over an exposure of the pulp of a tooth. (3)

Capsule, brain The bones surrounding and protecting the brain.

Caries The molecular decay or death of a bone, in which it becomes softened, discolored, and porous. It produces a chronic inflammation of the periosteum and surrounding tissues, and forms a cold abscess filled with a cheesy, fetid, puslike liquid, which generally burrows through the soft parts until it opens externally by a sinus or fistula. (2)

Caries, dental A disease of the calcified tissues of the teeth resulting from the action of microorganisms on carbohydrates, characterized by a decalcification of the inorganic portions of the tooth and accompanied or followed by disintegration of the organic portion. (2)

Cariogenic Conducive to caries. (2)

Carious Affected with or of the nature of caries. (2)

Cartilage A specialized, fibrous connective tissue, forming most of the temporary skeleton of the embryo, providing a model in which most of the bones develop, and constituting an important part of the growth mechanism of the organism. (2)

Cassette A radiographic plate holder.

Cementoblast A large cuboidal cell with spheroid or ovoid nucleus, found on the surface of cementum between the fibers, which is active in the formation of cementum. (2)

Cementoclast Cells which resorb cementum.

Cementocyte The cell found within lacunae of cellular cementum that possesses protoplasmic processes that course through the canaliculi of the cementum; derived from cementoblasts trapped within newly formed cementum.

Cementoenamel junction See *Junction cementoenamel*.
Cementum A specialized, calcified connective tissue that covers the anatomic root of a tooth.
Cephalometrics A scientific study of the measurements of the head.
Cephalometry Scientific measurement of the dimensions of the head. (2)
Cervix, n. Neck. The portion of the crown of the tooth near its junction with the root. (3)
Chromatin The more readily stainable portion of the cell nucleus, forming a network of nuclear fibrils within the achromatin of a cell. It is deoxyribose nucleic acid attached to a protein structure base and is the carrier of the genes in inheritance. Called also *chromoplasm*. (2)
Chromosome One of several small dark-staining more or less rod-shaped bodies which appear in the nucleus of a cell at the time of cell division. It contains the genes, or hereditary factors. The number of chromosomes in each species. The normal number in man is 46, with 22 pairs of autosomes and 2 sex chromosomes (XX or XY). (2)
Cicatrix A scar; the new tissue which is formed in the healing of a wound. (2)
Cleft lip A congenital cleft or defect in the upper lip, usually due to failure of the median nasal and maxillary processes to unite. The upper jaw or maxilla and palate may also be involved. (2)
Cleft palate See *Palate, cleft*.
Cohesive Uniting together, or characterized by cohesion. In dentistry, a property of annealed gold (foil or crystal) which causes separate particles to stick to one another, as they are welded, when placed in contact by heavy hand or mallet pressure. (3)
Colloid A translucent, yellowish, homogenous material of the consistency of glue, found in the cells and tissues in a state of colloid degeneration. A substance slowly diffusible, rather than soluble, in water and capable of passing through an animal membrane. (3)
Compound See *Dental compound*.
Compressive strength See *Strength, crushing*.
Condyle A rounded projection on a bone, usually for articulation with another bone. (2)
Congenital Present at birth and usually developed in utero. (1)
Contact points See *Point, contact*.
Crevice A narrow opening resulting from the separation of a junction.
Crevice, gingival The space between the gingiva and the enamel of the tooth crown; or in cases in which the gingiva has receded, between the gingiva and the cementum. (3)
Crown That portion of a tooth which is covered with enamel, and which projects from the tissues in which the root is fixed. (3)
Crushing strength See *Strength, crushing*.
Curettage Scraping or cleaning with a curette. (1)
Curette A surgical instrument having a sharp, spoon-shaped working blade; used for debridement. (1)
Cusp A pronounced elevation, or point, on the surface of a tooth, more especially on the occlusal surface. (3)
Cyst An abnormal cavity containing fluid or semifluid material, and, in the oral regions, almost always lined with epithelium. (1)

Deciduous See *Teeth, deciduous*.
Dental caries See *Caries, dental*.
Dental compound or compound A nonelastic molding or impression material that softens when heated and solidifies without a chemical change when cooled, i.e., thermoplastic.
Denticle A calcified body found in the pulp chamber of a tooth; it is composed either of irregular dentin (denticle) or it may be confused with an ectopic calcification of pulp tissue (false denticle). (1)
Dentin The portion of the tooth that lies subjacent to the enamel and cementum. Consists of an organic matrix upon which mineral salts are deposited; pierced by tubules containing filamentous protoplasmic processes of the odontoblasts that line the pulpal chamber and canal. It is of mesodermal origin. (1)
Dentin, primary The dentin formed before the eruption of a tooth. (2)
Dentin, secondary New dentin formed in response to stimuli associated with the normal aging process or with pathological conditions such as caries or injury, or cavity preparation; such dentin is highly irregular in nature. (2)
Dentinocemental junction See *Junction, dentinocemental*.
Dentition The teeth in the dental arch; ordinarily used to designate the natural teeth in position in their alveoli. (2)
Dentition, deciduous The 20 teeth which erupt first and are later replaced by the permanent teeth. (2)
Dentition, mixed The complement of teeth in the jaws after eruption of some of the permanent teeth, before all of the deciduous teeth are shed. (2)
Dentition, permanent The 32 teeth which erupt after the deciduous teeth are lost. (2)
Deposits, calcareous (tartar) (calculus) A concretion deposited on the teeth composed of calcium phosphate, calcium carbonate, magnesium phosphate, and other elements within an organic matrix composed of desquamated epithelium, mucin, microorganisms, and other debris. (1)
Development Gradual growth or expansion, especially from a lower to a higher stage of complexity.
Diagnosis The process by which one recognizes or identifies any condition that may be a departure from normal. (1)
Diapedesis The outward passage through intact vessel walls of corpuscular elements of the blood. (2)
Disc See *Disk*.
Disease(s) A definite morbid process having a characteristic train of symptoms; it may affect the whole body or any of its parts, and its etiology, pathology, and prognosis may be known or unknown. (2)
Disk A circular or rounded flat plate or organ.
Distal Away from the median line of the face following the curve of the dental arch. The surfaces of the teeth most distant from the median line are called distal surfaces. (3)
DNA deoxyribonucleic acid See *Acid, deoxyribonucleic*.
Duct A passage with well-defined walls; especially a tube for the passage of excretions or secretions. (2)
Ecology The study of the environment and life history of organisms. (2)
Ectoderm The outermost of the three primary germ layers of the embryo. From it are developed the epi-

dermis and the epidermal tissues, such as the nails, hair, and glands of the skin, the nervous system, the external sense organs, as the ear, eye, etc., and the mucous membrane of the mouth and anus. (2)

Edentulous Without teeth; lacking teeth.

Elastic Susceptible of being stretched, compressed, or distorted, and then tending to assume its original shape. (2)

Elastic limit See *Proportional limit.*

Elasticity The quality or condition of being elastic. (2)

Embryo(s) The early or developing stage of any organism, especially the developing product of fertilization of an egg. In the human, the embryo is generally considered to be the developing organism from one week after conception to the end of the second month. (2)

Eminence, articular A transverse bony ridge which, structurally speaking, is regarded as the medial root of the cheekbone or zygomatic arch. It is strongly convex in an anteroposterior direction and somewhat concave in a transverse direction. Medial and lateral borders are accentuated by fine bony ridges.

Enamel The vitreous covering tissue of the anatomic crowns of the teeth; consists of enamel rods, or prisms, and a cementing interrod substance. It is cleavable along the general direction of the rods.

Enamel, lamellae Thin dark bands visible in ground sections of teeth viewed with transmitted light; they extend through the entire thickness of the enamel and are thought to be organic matter or light-absorbing cracks. (2)

Enamel, mottled A defect in the enamel structure of the teeth which may be chalky white in color or yellow, brown or black. The enamel may be pitted. The discolored areas and pits may be of various sizes and degrees depending on the severity of the causative factor.

Enamel rods See *Rods, enamel.*

Enamel tufts See *Tufts, enamel.*

Endochondral Situated, formed, or occurring within cartilage. (2)

Entoderm or endoderm The innermost of the three primary germ layers of the embryo. From it are derived the epithelium of the pharynx, respiratory tract (except the nose), the digestive tract, bladder and urethra. (2)

Enzyme A protein substance which is a catalyst that speeds up metabolic and other processes involving organic materials. Some enzymes function within cells; others function in the extracellular fluids and tissue spaces and organs. They are active in all major tissue functions, such as cellular respiration, muscle contraction, digestive processes, and energy consumption, and are produced intracellularly. (1)

Epigenesis The theory that development starts from a structureless cell, and consists in the successive formation and addition of new parts which do not preexist in the fertilized egg: opposed to the theory of preformation. (2)

Epiglottis An elastic cartilage covered by mucous membrane that forms the superior part of the larynx and guards the glottis during swallowing. (1)

Epithelium The covering of internal and external surfaces of the body, including the lining of vessels and other small cavities. It consists of cells joined by small amounts of cementing substances. Epithelium is classified into types on the basis of the number of layers deep and the shape of the superficial cells. (2)

Epulis A tumor upon the gingiva.

Erosion, dental The wearing away or loss of tooth structure by chemical process without known bacterial action, beginning usually in the enamel at the neck of the tooth.

Erythrocyte (red blood cell) A yellowish, circular, biconcave disk, found in the blood, which contains hemoglobin and carries oxygen. In man they are about 7.7μ in diameter and about 1μ thick. There are normally about five million in each cubic millimeter of blood. (2)

Etiology The study or theory of the causation of any disease; the sum of knowledge regarding causes. (2)

Exfoliation The shedding of necrotic bone or dead epidermis. In dentistry, the physiologic loss of the deciduous dentition.

Exogenous Growing by additions to the outside; developed or originating outside the organism. (2)

Extension for prevention, dental Extending the margins of a cavity preparation to remove incipient carious lesions or to areas of the tooth that are either self-cleansing or readily cleansed. Such extensions are to prevent the recurrence of caries at the margins of the restoration.

Fauces The passage from the mouth to the pharynx, including both the lumen and its boundaries. (2)

Fetus The unborn offspring of any viviparous animal; the developing young in the human uterus after the end of the second month. Before 8 weeks it is called an embryo; it becomes an infant when it is completely outside the body of the mother, even before the cord is cut. (2)

Fiber An elongated, threadlike structure of organic tissue. (2)

Fiber(s), Sharpey's The collagenous extensions of the periodontal membrane fibers into the cementum and into the alveolar bone proper.

Fibroblasts Connective tissue cells which form the fibrous tissues of the body such as the tendons, aponeuroses, supporting and binding tissues. (2)

Fissure Any cleft or groove, normal or otherwise. In dentistry, a fault in the surface of a tooth caused by the imperfect joining of the enamel of the different lobes. To be distinguished from a groove or sulcus.

Fluorescence The property of emitting light after exposure to light, the wavelength of the emitted light being longer than that of the light absorbed. (2)

Fluoridation The addition of fluoride to the public water supply to help reduce the incidence of dental caries. (2)

Fluoride A binary compound of fluorine. (2)

Fluoridization The application of fluoride solution to the teeth. (2)

Fluorine A nonmetallic, gaseous element, belonging to the halogen group; symbol, F; atomic number, 9; atomic weight, 18.998. (2)

Foil Metal in the form of an extremely thin, pliable sheet. (2)

Foil, gold Pure gold rolled into an extremely thin sheet, used in the restoration of carious or fractured teeth. (2)

Follicle(s) A very small excretory or secretory sac or gland. (2)

Follicle, dental The structure within the substance of

the jaws enclosing the tooth before its eruption; the dental sac and its contents. (2)

Fontanelle(s) A soft spot, such as one of the membrane-covered spaces remaining in the incompletely ossified skull. (2)

Foramen A natural opening in a bone or other structure.

Foramen, apical An aperture at or near the apex of the root of a tooth, giving passage to the blood vessels and nerves supplying the pulp. (2)

Foramen, mandibular The opening on the medial aspect of the vertical ramus of the lower jaw or mandible approximately midway between the mandibular and gonial notches; may be located posterior to the middle of the ramus. It contains inferior alveolar vessels and the inferior alveolar nerve.

Foramen, mental A circular opening on the lateral aspect of the body of the lower jaw or mandible either below the apex of the first premolar or below the apex of the second premolar but usually between the first and second premolars inferior to their apices. The mental vessels and nerve pass through this foramen to supply the lip.

Fossa A pit, hollow, depression.

Fossa, dental A round, or angular depression in the surface of a tooth. Fossae occur mostly in the occlusal surfaces of the molars, and in the lingual surfaces of the incisors. (3)

Frontotemporal Pertaining to the frontal and temporal bones. (2)

Gel A solidified jellylike colloid. (3)

Gene The biologic unit of heredity, self-producing and located in a definite position (locus) on a particular chromosome. (2)

Genetic Pertaining to reproduction, or to birth or origin. Inherited. (2)

Gingiva The gum; the fibrous tissue, covered by mucous membrane which covers the alveolar processes of the upper and lower jaws and surrounds the necks of the teeth. (2)

Gingival crevice See *Crevice, gingival.*

Gingivectomy The surgical excision of unsupported gingival tissue to the level where it is attached, creating a new gingival margin apical in position to the old. (1)

Gingivitis Inflammation of the gingiva. See also ulitis. The term "gingivitis" should be limited to inflammation of the soft tissues immediately about the teeth and covering the borders of the alveolar processes, the term "ulitis" includes the wider inflammations that include the roof of the mouth and other parts. (3)

Gingivoplasty The surgical contouring of the gingival tissue in order to secure the physiologic architectural form necessary for the maintenance of tissue health and integrity. (1)

Glabella The most anterior point on the brain capsule on the midsagittal plane between the superciliary arches. In the living it is found above the root of the nose and between the median ends of the eyebrows.

Gland(s) An organ producing a specific product or secretion.

Globulin A class of proteins characterized by being insoluble in pure water but soluble in dilute salt solutions that occur widely in plant and animal tissues. (Webster)

Glottis The vocal apparatus of the larynx, consisting of the true vocal cords (vocal folds) and the opening between them (rima glottidis). (2)

Gnathion The lowest point of the lower jaw or mandible in the midline.

Gold, alloy See *Alloy, gold, dental.*

Gold, cohesive Gold in the form of foil or crystals, the surfaces of which are clean and free from condensed gases or salts so that they may be brought into actual contact. Gold foil or crystals in which the welding property is partially or fully developed. (3)

Gold foil See *Foil, gold.*

Gonion The apex or the point of maximum curvature at the mandibular angle.

Granuloma A tumor or neoplasm made up of granulation tissue (Virchow). (2)

Granuloma, dental A mass of granulation tissue usually surrounded by a fibrous sac continuous with the periodontal membrane and attached to the apex of a root; thought to be the result of a chronic periapical abscess. (2)

Groove A linear channel or sulcus, especially on the surface of a tooth. See also Sulcus. (2)

Growth (1) A normal process of increase in size, produced by accretion of tissue of a constitution similar to that originally present. (2) An abnormal formation, such as a tumor. (2)

Gums See *Gingiva.*

Gutta-percha A product of the latex or exudate from a tree of the family *Sapotaceae*. (3)

Hairlip See *Cleft lip.*

Haversian bone See *Bone, haversian.*

Haversian canal See *Canal, haversian.*

Haversian system See *System, haversian.*

Heredity The inheritance of resemblance, physical qualities, or diseases from a familial predecessor; the passage of characteristics from one generation to its progeny by genetic linkage. (1)

Histocyte A large phagocytic interstitial cell forming part of the reticulo-endothelial system. (2)

Horn of the pulp That part of the pulp tissue which extends toward the cusp of a tooth.

Impression, dental An imprint or negative likeness of the structures of the oral cavity from which a positive reproduction of the mouth may be made. (1)

Incidence, dental The amount of a dental disease that occurs during a specified period of time (usually a year).

Infection, primary focus of The original site of infection, which may result in a secondary manifestation of disease elsewhere in the body. (3)

Inion The crossing point of the midline on the brain capsule with a tangent to the upper convexities of the superior nuchal lines. It can be determined in the living with some degree of accuracy.

Inlay A porcelain or metal restoration to be inserted in a previously prepared cavity in a tooth and retained by cement. (3)

Inorganic Not of organic origin. Pertaining to substances not of organic origin. (2)

Interdentale, inferior The midline point in the facial part of the skull on the tip of the alveolar septum between the right and left lower central incisors.

Interdentale, superior The midline point in the facial part of the skull on the tip of the septum between the right and left upper central incisors.

Interproximal Between adjoining surfaces. The space between adjoining teeth as they stand in the line of the arch. (3)

Investment The material in which a denture, tooth, crown, or pattern for a dental restoration is enclosed before curing, soldering, or casting, or the process of enclosing it in such material. (2)

In vitro Within a glass; observable in a test tube. (2)

In vivo Within the living body. (2)

Isthmus A narrow connection between two larger bodies or parts; used as a general term to designate a connecting structure or region.

Joint The place of union between two or more bones of the skeleton. Also called an articulation.

Joint, temporomandibular The joint formed by the mandibular condyle of the lower jaw and the glenoid fossa of the skull. It is a sliding hinge joint. It is paired, and the joints act alternately as axes of rotation for each other. Each joint limits the range of motion of the other. The sliding or translatory action of the joint, coupled with both horizontal and vertical rotation, permits the mandible and its associated structures to move over a considerable volume of space during function.

Junction, cementoenamel The junction of the enamel of the crown and the cementum of the root of a tooth.

Junction, dentinocemental The line of union between the cementum and dentin on the root of a tooth.

Knoop Hardness Number A means of measuring the surface hardness of a material. A diamond indenting tool is used and the hardness determined by measuring the length of the indentation. The higher the number, the harder the material.

Labial Pertaining to the lips. Toward the lips. (3)

Labio-lingual From the lips toward the tongue; as the labio-lingual diameter of the central incisor. (3)

Lambda The point on the brain capsule at which sagittal and lamboid sutures meet.

Lamella A thin leaf or plate, as of bone. (2)

Lamella(e), enamel Microscopic faults in the enamel which extend inward from the surface of the tooth. They are filled with organic material and may form an entrance for caries-producing bacteria.

Lamella, haversian One of the concentric bony plates surrounding a haversian canal. (2)

Landmark An anatomic structure which is used as a guide in locating another structure or organ.

Landmark, cephalometric Points located on oriented head radiographs from which lines, planes, and angles may be constructed in order to analyze the configuration and relationship of elements of the cranial and facial skeleton.

Leukocyte (white blood cell) Any colorless, ameboid cell mass. Applied especially to one of the formed elements of the blood, consisting of a colorless granular mass of protoplasm, having ameboid movements, and varying in size between 0.005 and 0.015 mm. in diameter. (2)

Ligament, periodontal The fibrous tissue that surrounds the root of the tooth and connects the cementum of the tooth to the alveolar bone thereby holding the tooth in place.

Lingual Next to, or toward the tongue; as lingual surface of a tooth.

Lip, cleft See *Cleft lip.*

Luminescence The property of giving off light without showing a corresponding degree of heat. (2)

Lymphatic(s) Pertaining to or containing lymph, a transparent body fluid; by extension, the term is sometimes used alone to designate a lymphatic vessel. (2)

Malocclusion Such contact of the upper or maxillary and lower or mandibular teeth as will interfere with the highest efficiency during the excursive movements of the jaw that are essential to mastication; graded by Angle into four classes, depending on the degree of abnormality of the relationship. (2)

Mandible The horseshoe-shaped bone forming the lower jaw; the largest and strongest bone of the face, presenting a body and a pair of rami, which articulate with the skull at the temporomandibular joints. (2)

Marrow The soft material that fills the cavities of the bones. (2)

Mastication The process of chewing food in preparation for swallowing and digestion.

Matrix A mold in which anything is formed. A thin sheet of metal closely fastened on a tooth to form a fourth surrounding wall of a proximal cavity in a tooth. (3)

Maturation The stage or process of becoming mature. In biology, a process of cell division during which the number of chromosomes in the germ cells is reduced to one-half the number characteristic of the species. (2)

Maxilla The irregularly shaped bone that with its fellow forms the upper jaw; it assists in the formation of the eye socket or orbit, the nasal cavity, and the palate, and lodges the upper teeth. (2) See also *Process, maxillary.*

Median line The anterior-posterior perpendicular central line of the body. (3)

Mesial Toward the median line. Those surfaces of the teeth which, as they stand in the arch, and following its curve, are toward the median line, are called mesial surfaces. (3)

Mesio-distal From mesial to distal; as, the mesio-distal diameter of the lower first molar. (3)

Mesoderm The middle layer of the three primary germ layers of the embryo, lying between the ectoderm and the entoderm. From it are derived the connective tissue, bone and cartilage, the muscles, the blood and blood vessels, lymphatics and lymphoid organs, the notochord, the epithelium of pleura, pericardium, peritoneum, kidney and sex organs. (2)

Micron A unit of linear measure in the metric system, being 10^{-3} millimeter, or 10^{-6} meter. Abbreviated μ. mm.

Microscope An instrument which is used to obtain an enlarged image of small objects and to reveal details of structure not otherwise distinguishable. (2)

Microscope, electron An instrument in which an electron beam, instead of light, forms an image for viewing on a fluorescent screen, or for photography. (2)

Mitosis A method of indirect (nonsexual) division of a cell, consisting of a complex of various processes, by means of which the two daughter nuclei normally receive identical complements of the number of chromosomes characteristic of the somatic cells of the species. (2)

Model A positive, or duplicate, of the mouth structures, or some portion of them. (3)

Modulus of elasticity A measure of the stiffness of a material. It is obtained by dividing the stress below the proportional limit by the corresponding strain value. Often referred to as Youngs' Modulus.

Modulus of resilience See *Resilience*.

Mold A form in which an object is cast or shaped. The process of shaping a material into an object. The term used to specify the shape of an artificial tooth or teeth. (1)

Molecule A very small mass of matter; an aggregation of atoms; specifically, a chemical combination of two or more atoms which form a specific chemical substance. To break up the molecule into its constituent atoms is to change its character. The number of atoms in a molecule varies with the compound. (2)

Morphology The science of the forms and structures of organized beings.

Mottled teeth See *Teeth, mottled*.

Mucin An albuminoid substance, the chief constituent of mucus. It is insoluble in water and is precipitated by alcohol, alum and acids. Mucin is present in saliva, mucous secretions, the bile, and in certain cysts. (3)

Mucopolysaccharide A group of polysaccharides which contains hexosamine, which may or may not be combined with protein and which, dispersed in water, form many of the mucins. (2)

Mucosa, oral Lining of the oral cavity.

Mucus The free secretion of glands of mucous membranes, composed of mucin, and various inorganic salts, desquamated cells and leukocytes.

Muscle(s) An organ that, by cellular contraction, produces movements.

Muscle(s), facial The muscles of expression, frequently called the mimetic muscles. They are quite variable in contour, are widely distributed over the scalp and face, and tend to be especially concentrated about the orbits, the outer ear, and the lips. (1)

Muscle(s), masticatory The powerful muscles that elevate and rotate the mandible so that the opposing teeth may occlude for mastication.

Nasal septum See *Septum, nasal*.

Nasion The point in the skull where internasal and nasofrontal sutures meet.

Nasospinale The point in the head at which a line tangent to the lower margins of the nasal aperture is intersected by the midsagittal plane. (2)

Neck, dental That portion of the tooth which forms the junction of the crown and root. This term has been loosely applied. (3)

Necrosis Death of tissue, usually as individual cells, groups of cells, or in small localized areas. (2)

Neoplasm Any new and abnormal growth such as a tumor.

Nerve(s) A cordlike structure that conveys impulses from one part of the body to another.

Nerve, trigeminal The trigeminal nerve (fifth cranial nerve) is a mixed motor and sensory nerve composed of two components that leave the pons separately.

Notochord The rod-shaped body, composed of cells derived from the mesoblast, below the primitive groove of the embryo, defining the primitive axis of the body. (2)

Nutrition The process of assimilating food. Nutriment. (2)

Occlusal surface See *Surface, occlusal*.

Occlusion, abnormal See *Malocclusion*.

Occlusion, centric The relation of the upper to the lower teeth when the jaws are closed and at rest. (3)

Occlusion, dental The relation of the maxillary and mandibular teeth when in functional contact during activity of the mandible. (2) See also *Malocclusion*.

Occlusion, normal The normal contact of the teeth of the lower jaw with those of the upper when the mouth is closed. (3)

Odontoblast(s) Connective tissue cells that line the surface of the dental pulp adjacent to the dentin. During the tooth development period they have much to do with the formation of dentin. (2)

Odontoclast(s) A multinucleated giant cell (osteoclast), found associated with absorption of the roots of a deciduous tooth. (2)

Ohm The electric resistance of a column of mercury for 1 square millimeter in cross section and 106 centimeters long; the unit of electric resistance. (2)

Opisthion The midline point on the brain capsule at the posterior border of the occipital foramen.

Orale The point of the end of the incisive suture on the inner surface of the alveolar process. (2)

Orbitale The lowest point of the infraorbital margin in the facial part of the skull.

Organic Having an organized structure. Pertaining to substances derived from living organisms. (2)

Orthodontics That branch of dentistry which deals with the prevention and correction of irregularities of the teeth and malocclusion, and with associated facial problems. (2)

Ossification The formation of bone or of a bony substance; the conversion of fibrous tissue or of cartilage into bone or a bony substance. (2)

Osteoblast(s) The cells which form bone. (3)

Osteoclast(s) Cells which are concerned with the absorption and removal of bone.

Osteogenesis Formation of bone; the development of the bones. (2)

Overbite The overlapping of mandibular or lower incisor teeth by the upper maxillary incisor teeth. (1)

Palate The roof of the mouth. It consists of a hard anterior part (the hard palate) and a soft movable part (the soft palate).

Palate, cleft A palate having a congenital fissure in the median line. (2)

Papilla(e) A small, nipple-shaped projection or elevation.

Papilla, dental The enlargement at the base of a dental follicle from which the dentin of a tooth is developed.

Pathogen Any disease-producing microorganism or material. (2)

Pearl, epithelial A discrete, rounded or ovid mass (frequently ranging from 30 to 150μ in diameter) that consists of keratin in which fairly well differentiated, neoplastic squamous cells are arranged in a whorled or concentrically laminated pattern, with polygonal cells in the central portion and flattened; more mature cells peripherally. Termed also epithelial nest. (4)

Pedodontics The department of dentistry which is concerned with the diagnosis and treatment of conditions of the teeth and mouth in children. (2)

Periapical Relating to tissues encompassing the apex of a tooth, including periodontal membrane and alveolar bone. (2)

Periodontal ligament See *Ligament, periodontal.*

Periodontics That branch of dentistry dealing with the study and treatment of periodontal diseases. (2)

Periodontitis Inflammation of the periodontium. (1)

Periodontium The tissues investing and supporting the teeth, including the cementum, periodontal membrane, alveolar bone, and gingiva. Anatomically, the term is restricted to the connective tissue interposed between the teeth and their bony sockets. (2)

Periodontosis A degenerative, noninflammatory condition of the periodontium, originating in one or more of the periodontal structures and characterized by destruction of the tissues. (2)

Pharynx The musculomembranous sac between the mouth and nares and the esophagus. It is a simple, funnel-shaped tube of muscle tissue that is wide at the head end and narrow at the esophageal end. It is the common pathway for the air and food passages; food cannot be long retained there but must be either passed down to the esophagus or regurgitated back into the mouth.

Phosphorescence The emission of light without appreciable heat; the property of continuing luminous in the dark after exposure to light or other radiation. (2)

Pit, dental A sharp, pointed depression in the enamel. Pits occur mostly where several developmental grooves join; as in the occlusal surfaces of the molars, at the endings of the buccal grooves on the buccal surfaces of the molars; occasionally in the lingual surfaces of the incisors. (3)

Plaque, bacterial A deposit of material upon the surface of a tooth which acts as a medium for the lodgment and growth of bacteria, causing dental caries. (2)

Plaster of paris The hemihydrate of calcium sulfate that, when mixed with water, forms a paste which subsequently sets into a hard mass. (1)

Pocket A saclike space or cavity.

Pocket, periodontal A pathologic deepening of the gingival sulcus produced by destruction of the supporting tissues and apical proliferation of the epithelial attachment. Ulceration of the pocket epithelium lining is characteristic. Also called gingival pocket. (1)

Point, contact The point on the proximal surface of a tooth which touches a neighboring tooth. (3)

Polysaccharide One of a group of carbohydrates which contain more than four molecules of simple carbohydrates combined with each other. They comprise the dextrins, starches and glycogen; also cellulose, gums, inulin and pectose. (2)

Porion A cephalometric landmark, being the midpoint on the upper edge of the porus acusticus externus, situated about 5 mm. above the superior margin of the cutaneous external auditory meatus. (2)

Precancerous Pertaining to an early stage in the development of cancer. (2)

Precursor A substance from which another substance is formed.

Prevalence The number of cases of a disease in existence at a certain time in a designated area. (2)

Prevention, extension for See *Extension for prevention.*

Primary focus of infection See *Infection, primary focus of.*

Process In anatomy, a marked prominence or projection of a bone. In dentistry, a series of operations that convert a wax pattern of a dental appliance into a permanent restoration composed of some relatively indestructible material.

Process, alveolar The part of the bone that surrounds and supports the teeth in the maxilla and the mandible.

Process, condyloid The posterior process on the ramus of the mandible that articulates with the mandibular fossa of the temporal bone. (2)

Process, coronoid The anterior part of the upper end of the ramus of the mandible, to which the temporal muscle is attached. (2)

Process, maxillary The irregularly shaped bone forming one-half of the upper jaw. The upper jaw is made up of the two maxillae. (1)

Process, palatine One of four shelflike extensions of the embryonic upper jaw that give rest to the premaxillary palate and palate.

Procreation The entire process of bringing a new individual into the world.

Prognathism The projection or abnormal growth of the jaws. (1)

Prognosis A forecast as to the probable result of an attack of disease; the prospect as to recovery from a disease as indicated by the nature and symptoms of the case. (2)

Prognosis, dental An evaluation of the results to be achieved from treatment of certain conditions of the mouth, or from the use of dental prostheses. (2)

Proliferation Growth by reproduction of similar cells.

Prophylactic A remedy that tends to ward off disease. (1)

Prophylaxis Preventive medicine.

Prophylaxis, oral Preventive measures against diseases of the mouth. (3)

Proportional limit The maximal stress to which a material may be subjected and still be capable of returning to its original dimension when the force is released. This stress at which permanent deformation first occurs may be referred to as the elastic limit.

Prosthesis The replacement of an absent part of the human body by an artificial part. (1)

Prosthesis, dental An artificial replacement for one or more natural teeth or associated structures. (1)

Prosthodontics That branch of dental art and science concerned with the construction of artificial appliances designed to replace missing teeth and sometimes other parts of the oral cavity and face. (2)

Protrusion To thrust forward, as the protrusive movement of the mandible in biting. (3)

Proximal That surface of a tooth that is toward, nearest, or in contact with another tooth to the mesial or distal as the teeth are arranged in the arch. (3)

Pulp chamber The central opening in the dentin of the crown portion of a tooth which is occupied by the pulp of the tooth. In the double and triple-rooted teeth, the pulp chambers are very distinct from the root canals, but in teeth having but one root the pulp chamber is not distinctly divided from the root canal. (3)

Pulp, dental The highly vascular connective tissue contained within the pulp cavity of a tooth; made up of gelatinous ground substance, collagenous and argyrophilic fibers, cellular elements, terminal blood vessels, lymph vessels, and nerves.

Pulpectomy The extirpation of the pulp from the pulp chamber and root canals of a tooth. (2)

Pulpitis Inflammation of the dental pulp. (2)

Pulpotomy The surgical excision of the coronal portion of a vital tooth pulp. (2)

Pyorrhea Obsolete term for periodontitis. See *Periodontitis*.

Radiogram See *Radiograph*.

Radiograph A film or other record produced by the action of actinic rays on a sensitized surface, such as an autoradiogram, or a roentgenogram. (2)

Radiolucent Permitting the passage of radiant energy, yet offering some resistance to it. (2)

Radiopaque Opaque to the roentgen ray; not permitting the passage of radiant energy. (2)

Ramus, mandibular The ascending portion of the lower jawbone.

Resilience The amount of energy which may be absorbed by a material before the proportional limit is exceeded. Usually measured by the modulus of resilience which is the amount of energy stores in a material when one unit volume is stressed to the proportional limit.

Resorption The loss of substance through physiologic or pathologic means, such as the loss of dentin and cementum of a tooth, or of the alveolar process of the mandible or maxilla. (2)

Restoration, dental A broad term applied to any inlay, crown, bridge, partial denture, or complete denture that restores or replaces loss of tooth structure, teeth, or oral tissues. (1)

Rods, enamel A calcified column or prism, with an average diameter of 4 mm.; extends in a wavy pattern through the entire thickness of the enamel; generally is perpendicular to the surface of the tooth. (1)

Root That portion of the tooth that is fixed in the alveolus, or socket, and is covered with cementum. (3)

Root canal See *Canal, root*.

Rubber dam A thin sheet of very elastic rubber used for keeping the teeth, and especially cavities in the teeth, dry and clean while performing such operations as filling, removing pulps, filling pulp (root) canals, etc.

Rugae, dental A series of irregular ridges in the hard palate of the mouth.

Saliva The clear, slightly acid mucoserous secretion formed in the parotid, submandibular, sublingual, and smaller oral mucous glands. It has lubricative, cleansing, bactericidal, excretory, and digestive functions and is also an aid to swallowing or deglutition.

Scaler An instrument designed to be used in removing deposits, particularly calculus, from the teeth.

Sella turcica The center of the pituitary fossa of the sphenoid bone.

Septum, nasal The thin, vertical bony septum separating the right and left nasal cavities. (1)

Sharpey's fibers See *Fibers, Sharpey's*.

Silica The purest of three major ingredients that make up dental porcelain. It imparts stiffness and hardness to the product and is the framework around which the kaolin and feldspar contract. (1)

Skeleton The bony framework of the body; in vertebrate animals, the bones of the body collectively.

Skeleton, facial The bony framework of the anterior aspect of the head from the forehead to the chin inclusive.

Socket A hollow or depression, into which a corresponding part fits. (2)

Socket, dry A condition sometimes occurring after tooth extraction, resulting in exposure of bone with localized osteomyelitis of an alveolar crypt, and symptoms of severe pain. (2)

Socket, tooth The dental alveoli, the cavities in the maxilla and mandible in which the teeth are embedded. (2)

Space maintainer An appliance used to prevent loss of space in the dental arch created by the premature loss of deciduous teeth.

Spatially Of or pertaining to space.

Spine, anterior nasal The small bony projection extending forward from the medial anterosuperior part of each maxilla.

Spine, posterior nasal The small, sharp bony point projecting backward from the midline of the horizontal part of the palatine bone.

Sprue (ingate) Wax or metal used to form the aperture or apertures through which a material such as gold or resin may enter a mold to make a casting; also the material that later fills the sprue hole or holes. (1)

Staphylion The midline point in the facial part of the skull of a line connecting the most anterior points of the posterior border of the hard palate on either side.

Sterile 1. Not fertile; infertile; barren; not producing young. 2. Aseptic; not producing microorganisms; free from microorganisms. (2)

Sterilize 1. To render sterile; to free from microorganisms. 2. To render incapable of reproduction. (2)

Strength, crushing (compressive strength) The greatest unit stress a body can sustain without rupture. (3)

Stress Forcibly exerted influence; pressure. In dentistry the pressure of the lower teeth against the upper in mastication.

Structure The components and their manner of arrangement in constituting a whole. (2)

Sulcus A furrow, trench, or groove, as on the surface of the brain or in folds of mucous membrane. A groove or depression on the surface of a tooth. A groove in a portion of the oral cavity. (1)

Surface(s), axial Those surfaces of the teeth that are parallel with their long axes. They are labial or buccal, lingual, mesial, and distal surfaces. (3)

Surface, buccal Toward the cheek.

Surface, distal Away from the median line of front center of the mouth.

Surface, incisal The cutting edge of the incisors and canines are sometimes called incisal surfaces. (3)

Surface, labial Toward the lip. (1)

Surface, lingual Toward the tongue. (1)

Surface, occlusal The grinding surface of the molar and premolar teeth.
Surface, proximal The surface of a tooth nearest the adjacent tooth.
Surface tension See *Tension, surface*.
Suture A type of fibrous joint in which the opposed surfaces are closely united. 2. A stitch or series of stitches made to secure apposition of the edges of a surgical or accidental wound; used also as a verb to indicate the application of such stitches. 3. Material used in closing a surgical or accidental wound with stitches. (2)
System, endocrine The system of glands which elaborate internal secretions, including the pituitary, parathyroid, thyroid, and suprarenal glands.
System, haversian A long, cylindrical region in bone, usually placed lengthwise of the long bones, composed of a central canal surrounded by a number of concentric rings or layers of bone corpuscles.
Tartar See *Deposits, calcareous*.
Teeth See *Tooth*.
Teeth, deciduous The first set of 20 teeth. Variously referred to as baby teeth, first teeth, primary teeth.
Teeth, mottled Marked with spots of different color or shades of color. blotched, variegated. (3)
Temporomandibular joint See *Joint, temporomandibular*.
Tensile strength (ultimate strength) The greatest unit of tensile stress which can be induced in a structure before rupture. (3)
Tension, surface A molecular force existing in the surface film of all liquids measured as force per unit length. (3)
The bite See *Bite*.
Tissue An aggregation of similarly specialized cells united in the performance of a particular function. (2)
Tissue, granulation Young vascularized connective tissue formed in the process of healing of ulcers and wounds and ultimately forming the cicatrix. (2)
Tissue, lymphoid A lattice work of reticular tissue the interspaces of which contain lymphocytes.
Tongue The movable, muscular organ on the floor of the mouth, subserving the special sense of taste and aiding in mastication, deglutition, and the articulation of sound. (2)
Tooth, teeth Principal organs of mastication.
Tooth, deciduous See *Dentition, deciduous*.
Tooth, permanent See *Dentition, permanent*.

Trabecula A little beam; used in anatomical nomenclature as a general term to designate a supporting or anchoring strand of connective tissue; for example, a strand extending from a capsule into the substance of the enclosed organ. (2)
Treatment The mode or course pursued for remedial ends.
Treatment, preventive That management and care of a patient in which the aim is to prevent the occurrence of the disease. (2)
Trigeminal nerve See *Nerve, trigeminal*.
Tubules, dental Minute channels in dentin, extending from the pulp cavity to the cement and enamel.
Tuft(s) A small clump or cluster; a coil.
Tufts, enamel Hypocalcified, brushlike ends of some enamel rods that occasionally extend from the dentinoenamel junction into the enamel.
Tumor A mass of new tissue which persists and grows independently of its surrounding structures and which has no physiologic use. (2)
Ulitis A general inflammation of the gums as distinguished from gingivitis, which is confined to the free margins of the gums and immediate neighborhood. (3)
Ultrastructure The structural arrangement of the ultramicrons in a tissue or of the organelles in a cell.
Uvula, palatine A pendent, fleshy mass hanging from the soft palate above the root of the tongue, composed of the levator and tensor palati muscles, the unpaired uvula muscles, connective tissue, and mucous membrane. (2)
Veins The blood vessels that conduct the blood from the capillary bed back to the heart. They range in increasing size from the venules, to the small veins, to the large veins. The venules are small veins which are of special clinical interest to the dentist.
Yield strength An approximation of the first marked deviation from direct proportionality between stress and strain. It is calculated from the stress-strain curve and is roughly comparable to the proportional limit and elastic limit. As for those values, it is a measure of the force required to produce permanent deformation in a material.
Youngs' modulus See *Modulus of elasticity*.
Zygion The most lateral projection in the facial part of the skull of the zygomatic arch.
Zygoma The zygomatic process of the temporal or cheek bone. (2)
Zygomaxillare The lowermost point of the zygomaticomaxillary suture in the facial part of the skull.

www.ingramcontent.com/pod-product-compliance
Lightning Source LLC
Chambersburg PA
CBHW081758300426
44116CB00014B/2162